The Country Doctor Revisited
A Twenty-First Century Reader
EDITED BY THERESE ZINK

Over the past thirty years, rural health care in the United States has changed dramatically. The stereotypical white-haired doctor with his black bag of instruments and his predominantly white, small-town clientele has imploded: the global age has reached rural America. Independently owned clinics have given way to a massive system of hospitals, new technology now brings specialists right to the patient's bedside, and an increasingly diverse clientele has sparked the need for doctors and nurses with an equally diverse assortment of skills.

The Country Doctor Revisited is a fascinating collection of essays, poems, and short stories written by rural health care professionals on the experiences of doctors and nurses practicing medicine in rural environments, such as farms, reservations, and migrant camps. The pieces explore the benefits and burdens of new technology, the dilemmas in making ethically sound decisions, and the trials of caring for patients in a broken system. Alternately compelling, thought provoking, and moving, they speak of the diversity of rural health care providers, the range of patients served in rural communities, the variety of settings that comprise the rural United States, and the resources and challenges health care providers and patients face today.

Compliments of
Southern Vermont Area Health
Education Center
and the Advanced MedQuest program
June 16-21, 2013

The Country Doctor Revisited

Literature and Medicine

MICHAEL BLACKIE, EDITOR

CAROL DONLEY AND MARTIN KOHN, FOUNDING EDITORS

The Country Doctor Revisited

A Twenty-First Century
Reader

Edited by Therese Zink

The Kent State

University Press

KENT, OHIO

Library of Congress Catalog Card Number 2010020020
ISBN 978-1-60635-061-4
Manufactured in the United States of America

Names and identifying information have been altered to protect the privacy of those who
inspired these stories, poems, and essays included in this collection.

LIBRARY OF CONGRESS CATALOGING-IN-PUBLICATION DATA
The country doctor revisited : a twenty-first century reader / edited by Therese Zink.
p.   cm. — (Literature and medicine series)
Includes bibliographical references.
ISBN 978-1-60635-061-4 (pbk. : alk. paper) ∞
1. Medicine, Rural—United States. I. Zink, Therese, 1955– II. Series: Literature and medicine (Kent, Ohio); 18. [DNLM: 1. Rural Health Services—United States—Collected Works.
2. Rural Health Services—United States—Personal Narratives. 3. Rural Health Services—
United States—Poetry. WA 390 C855 2010]
RA771.5.C68 2010
362.1'04257—dc22   2010020020

British Library Cataloging-in-Publication data are available.

14 13 12 11   5 4 3

Contents

Introduction

In this collection we hear the voices of men and women who provide care and facilitate healing in modern rural settings: doctors, midwives, psychologists, nurses, emergency medical responders, and students, as diverse in ethnicity, gender, and age as those they serve. These storytellers, essayists, and poets live in small towns across the rural United States. They marvel, grumble, cry, grapple, and meditate on the beauty and challenges they encounter in their healing practices.

Today, rural health care encompasses more than the black bag of instruments and all the knowledge the doctor has in his head en route to a house call in the middle of the night. The stereotype of an elderly white-haired doctor and his predominately white, small-town clientele has imploded. The global age has reached rural America. House calls still occur, but the physician usually has a PDA or iPhone in her black bag. Although bartering medical care for a sack of potatoes or a few chickens may still occur, more common are the morass of the payment system and the alphabet soup of regulations.

The waiting room is increasingly heterogeneous too. Growing populations of new Americans as well as undocumented workers populate small, rural towns and create more business on Main Street and with it unfamiliar shops. Health practitioners are forced to accommodate languages besides English and to develop processes that oblige different cultural needs and expectations. Longtime rural residents have aged, challenging communities to develop social supports like Meals on Wheels and other programs for their elders. Troubled by many of the same problems as metropolitan areas—poverty, mental illness, addiction, and violence—rural areas struggle because support services are limited and geographically more dispersed. Traditionally reclusive groups continue to reach out to an increasingly complex world for assistance with the health and life issues they cannot manage on their own.

Resources in rural America are enhanced and complicated by rapidly evolving telecommunication, computer, and air transport systems as well as expanding health care systems that link the mountains, hills, plains, and deserts with the high-tech services available at metro area hospitals. Patients and their families have more options for treatment and increased responsibility in managing their illnesses. These alternatives are often remarkably successful but are costly and raise numerous ethical issues as well.

Rural clinics must incorporate complex steps to run a lab test, request a CAT scan, and collect payment—all put into place to assure quality of care and privacy and to weed out fraudulent business practices. However, these procedures have made survival as a solo practitioner difficult and for many impossible. "The girl" at the front desk has become several people with a variety of certifications after their names, such as coding or billing specialist, claims or health information clerk, and transcription or medical records technician.

Practitioners are called to do what they do for many of the same reasons as the stereotypical country doctor, acting out of a genuine concern for the patients who come to them and with the excitement and satisfaction of solving problems. As members and leaders in their communities, and with less bureaucracy, these twenty-first century practitioners brainstorm and sometimes find creative solutions that can be models for others.

This reader is organized into four sections, each accompanied by a section synopsis: Who We Are, Where We Are, Whom We Serve, and Our Resources and Challenges. I hope these stories, essays, and poems will encourage reflection and provoke discussion. I trust they will inspire young men and women to learn more about being healers in rural communities, spend time with a practitioner to see what rural practice entails, and pursue the education to join the struggling labor force of rural health care practitioners. Ultimately, may the voices in this collection galvanize public opinion and affect policy that can improve health care delivery across the rural United States.

Who We Are

Who We Are—Synopsis

GODFREY ONIME

The yellow-, red-, and green-striped gift bag containing the present lay on my office desk among the stacks of charts and assorted papers. Curious as to the sender, I looked at the card that came with it. "Oh no, not again." It was from my patient Ms. Emalee, next on my schedule. Among her myriad medical problems—diabetes, hypertension, obstructive sleep apnea—was intractable knees and back pain for which she used narcotics chronically. On her current visit I'd planed to perform a random drug test, to ensure she was actually taking the medications and that she did not use illicit drugs. But now the gift, although this was far from her first—she often brought fruits, baked goods and other presents for everyone in my clinic. After she learned I got married and hinted she was looking for "something special" for me, I'd entreated her not to worry. She had looked at me as if I were from a different planet and then declared I was "like family now," adding "you better believe you getting something from me, don't matter you snucked off 'n' got married without telling no one." Now I wondered: What if her test results indicated a problem? Would her act of kindness make it difficult for me to do my job, such as refusing to prescribe further narcotics or even discharging her from my practice?

The question of boundaries with their patients is one issue that small-town doctors face. Often for lack of convenient alternatives, country doctors not only have to take their friends on as patients, but their patients quickly establish themselves as friends. Given that the conventional medical ethics frowns on doctors treating friends or relatives, Dr. Kullnat grapples with this dilemma as it applies to rural medicine. In "Boundaries" she asks if a doctor could both be friends with their patients and be objective in caring for them. Dr. Farah's "LIFEprayerDEATH," manages to blur the boundary even further. It seems to challenge the reader to consider that in small towns, where privacy is shunned and familiarity with neighbors prized, maybe physicians' closeness with their patients is exactly what they need to render care with true understanding and deep compassion. This theme is further explored in Arne Vainio's "Mashkiki-winini: Thanking Sylvester for His Unconditional Smile" when the author cares for a patient with end-stage cancer and wrestles with the difficulty of accessing up-to-date diagnostics and treatments in a rural setting. Another essay, David McCray's "Three Days Changed My Grandfather's Life," seems to erase the boundary, when the author is confronted with a grandfather he adores and respects.

When I entered Ms. Emalee's room, she looked up at me expectantly and asked if I liked her present. I told her I had not opened it. Sensing her disappointment, I quickly added that I was waiting to get home, before opening it with my wife. The explanation seemed to satisfy her. "Smart man," she said, "I'm sure she'd love it." Ms. Emalee's knees and back still hurt, but her pain medications were helping. No, she did not have significant side effects from the medications, such as constipation or drowsiness. I also asked if she ever sold her pain pills, but that seemed to annoy her. "You keep asking me that foolish question every time I comes here and I keeps telling you no, I does not sells my medicines. Don't you even trust me?" I apologized, but reminded her it was the law and my job to ask. At the conclusion of the visit, I told her I'd like a sample of her urine for a random drug test. "Whatever you say, doc," was her sarcastic reply. Then she informed me they were having a birthday party for her mother—who was also my patient (as were her two sons, a daughter, a sister, and brother-in-law). Her mother was turning eighty. Her family would be greatly honored if my wife and I could come. Not sure how to respond, I promised to get back with her.

My early notions of the country doctor come from Norman Rockwell's 1954 painting "Doctor and Boy Looking at Thermometer" in which a kindly doctor making a house call sits on an unmade bed. The patient, a prepubescent boy, kneeling in bed, rests his head on the doctor's right shoulder as he peers with the doctor at the reading on the thermometer—an unmistakable indication of the bond between doctor and patient. Most people would agree that the idea that this image represents has been lost to today's fast-paced and complex world of medicine, where, as one patient complained of his previous doctor, a physician using an electronic medical record system may pay more attention to the computer than to making eye contact with patients. But besides technology, modern medicine is besieged with countless other intricacies that threaten the cosmopolitan as well as the country doctor—not the least of which are the effects of such acronyms as HMO and RVU and phrases like "risk management" and "pay for performance" discussed by Deborah Lee Luskin as she takes the reader through the struggle she and her husband had in their rural clinic. This is painfully obvious in Patricia J. Harman's "Teen Pregnancy," in which she, the nurse midwife, must explain to a pregnant sixteen-year-old that she and her family-physician husband no longer do deliveries because of the malpractice cost, which jumped from $70,000 to $130,000 per year. "You can buy a pretty good house in Jefferson County for that amount, a house every year, that's what it amounts to," she explains.

Thankfully, many physicians serving rural communities still manage to incorporate—if not hang on to—their Norman Rockwell image of the country doctor. In the process, they offer their patients expedient and excellent care, while learning a thing or two about themselves. Indeed, the reader cannot help being amused and intrigued by the experience of Dr. Gibes when he found himself clutching a steak knife while making a house call to an Amish family.

The landscape of today's rural medicine has changed in another significant respect: the faces of the doctors themselves. In Rockwell's "Doctor and Boy Looking at Thermometer," the physician is a white male. Today, that country doctor could just as easily be a woman—or even an Asian, African, or Hispanic, a far cry from the Rockwell painting. While these immigrants help to allay the manpower crunch in rural areas, the local people have to learn to understand them. But the physicians also face pressure of their own: that of fitting in. My own essay for this collection, "When Hostility Melted for the Funny Accent," examines my struggle to comprehend the people and the concept of family in my small, southern American town. Dr. Verghese, in his characteristic rich and elaborate style, even goes as far as exploring the challenges of alien doctors and their families independent of caring for patients. He and his Indian colleagues and families essentially formed their own subculture. In my mind, this adds to the richness of the place, just as a city like New York is no doubt enhanced by the endless ethnic and cultural diversity: Jews, Italians, Jamaicans, Indians, Chinese, gays, and lesbians. Diversity, I think, is the most rapid and sure road to development. I can attest that almost every foreign doctor in my local community felt comfortable enough settling in the area because they found someone like them here.

Other works in this section (Ann Floreen Niedringhaus and Richard Berlin) invoke the frustrations and joys of today's rural medicine. Another particularly stirring poem by Cinnamon Bradley calls for country doctors to be not just witnesses but participants in the living and dying of their patients. It invokes a place where "Everyone knew what Dr. Lee's clinic was for, but it was still a secret in this small Mississippi town," and where "people whispered laughter . . . as was appropriate." But Dr. Bradley "wanted to scream" for the country doctor to be different.

Was Dr. Kullnat's "Boundaries" a form of screaming too, a shout to the medical profession that one set of ethics does not suffice for all locales of medical practice, that technological and loan repayment requirements do not apply to all doctors equally? Perhaps these are some of the areas that need further work. I am also amazed at the number of cancellations and no-shows to my clinic, ostensibly for transportation needs. Are there ways of correcting these, or should there be provisions and assistance for the rural doctors to return to the days of Norman Rockwell, when house visits were a welcomed part of the profession?

The day that I received the present from Ms. Emalee, my wife and I unwrapped it once I was home. We erupted into laughter as soon as we saw it: the statuette of a bald African woman standing tall in a regal outfit. "I love it," my wife declared. "Tell her I just love it and thanks." She put it among our assorted collections on a shelf in the living room.

Ms. Emalee's urine drug screen showed she was using her narcotic medications and that she was not using illicit drugs. I called to tell her this, as she liked to be informed of all the results of her tests as soon as they become available. I also thanked her for the present. She reminded me about her mother's upcoming birthday party and the family's hope that I could attend. I remembered how we narrowly lost her mother at the hospital only months before, how I allowed Ms. Emalee's tears to stain my shirt when she feared the lump in her own breast may be cancer, how two years ago I prayed with the family at her brother's funeral, who was also my patient. Like many families, this one had seen its share of pain, and I felt honored being there for them. Now was their time to celebrate; I decided it was only proper I be a part of it.

That, in my mind, is what makes a complete country doctor—the image, I believe, that all the preceding essays help to illuminate.

LIFEprayerDEATH

KATHLEEN FARAH

"I prayed for you"

> she said.

"I prayed every day you would have a healthy baby."

> I did.

She sat across the aisle from me at church you know,
Exchanged greetings of peace and watched my pregnant belly grow.

> We prayed.

Tall in my white coat I stood before her in shivering snowflake gown.

My eyes and hands observed the tumor her right arm birthed had grown.

> I sighed.

Too few weeks later I kneel beside her in her home hospice bed.
"I pray for you"

> I silently said.

Words and tears are blocked by "professional boundaries" in my head.

> I silently cried.

"I pray you have a peaceful death."

> She did.

Boundaries

MEGAN WILLS KULLNAT

Some say that a delirious patient is unaware of the situation around him. That may be true. But as I peered into my patient's face, I saw clarity in his venerable eyes. And terror. Smiling down at him reassuringly, I began to organize admission orders and formulate a plan for his care.

Out of the corner of my eye, I noticed an emergency department nurse crouched by his bedside, gripping his hand. Despite the cacophony of beeping monitors and intrusive voices, my attention was drawn to the compassion in her grasp, the concern in her furrowed brow. Immediately impressed by her bedside manner, I paused with my paperwork to watch her. Moments later, a tear trailed from her lower lash to her trembling lip. I had rarely seen such empathy at the university. My thoughts were interrupted by another staff person bellowing for morphine. The nurse mumbled something in response. When nobody reacted, she repeated more clearly, "He's allergic to morphine." Surprised, everyone turned to her. "I know," she sighed, "because he's my grandfather."

In the first few years of medical school, "dual relationships" are briefly addressed in ethics class. When it comes to patient relationships, physicians-in-training are advised to avoid treating family members or close friends. In fact, numerous medical associations advise that "professional objectivity may be compromised. . . . As a general rule it should be avoided." This had seemed common sense to me, prior to spending a five-week rotation in a rural community as required by my medical school curriculum. However, upon arriving at this small rural community, I took an immediate interest in dual relationships: they were everywhere I looked. Yet look as I might, I struggled to find how these ethical guidelines were applicable to such a community.

Can dual relationships be avoided in a small town? Should they even be avoided? During twenty-minute personal interviews, I queried nine physicians and nine patients in Tillamook. The former group included general practitioners, obstetrician/gynecologists, surgeons, and Emergency Department physicians. The patients were a diverse group, including nurses, a lawyer, an insurance agent, a barber, and a banker. I sat with the city commissioner in the courthouse, the

CEO/president of the hospital in his office, with a judge in the courtroom. What I found both surprised and intrigued me.

No one was familiar with the term dual relationships, nor with the aforementioned guidelines. Many reacted with shock, and most stated without hesitation, "That's not possible in a small town." In fact, only one of the patients denied having a dual relationship with his physician. This individual maintained that he preferred distance from his physician because he was concerned that they would begin discussing medicine outside the office. He did not identify other potential downfalls of a dual relationship. Of note, this patient was relatively new to town and acknowledged that he often felt like "the new guy" with other town residents.

The remaining patients professed a deep and mutually respectful relationship with their physician. In some cases, their physician had cared for their parents, and even grandparents, before them. Rather than feeling uncomfortable disclosing information issues because they knew their doctor outside the office, they were more at ease discussing sensitive issues because of their friendship. One noted, "Guys don't talk about emotional issues . . . but our friendship makes it easier. . . . I don't look forward to the day [my doctor] retires." When asked if he withholds any potentially embarrassing information, he stated, "If I am to fully utilize him as a doc, I can't withhold anything. I'm not the first person in his office. It may be very personal to me, but he's heard it a hundred times. He doesn't internalize it, so why should I?"

Similarly, another patient declared, "We put on a different hat when we're doing business." Also having benefited from a dual relationship, he finds that he can be more honest and candid with his physician because of their friendship. "I respect him too much to not be truthful." This patient, like many others, recognized that the advantages and disadvantages of dual relationships are closely linked. A disadvantage is that one loses anonymity and privacy. An advantage is that one is constantly reminded to improve one's health: "If I haven't followed up on something and I see my doc at a poker game, he'll bug me to come in and get checked!" This patient also emphasized that a friendship makes his physician feel more approachable and that, indeed, "The best doctors are warm, humane, and open."

Other patients echo the importance of a physician's ability to interact on a social level with the community. One noted, "It's almost impossible to separate the two worlds. Social situations reinforce trust and confidence. If you don't know your physician, how do you know you can trust him?" Another notes, "Doctors need to be seen as humans. There is an image that they are 'uppity.' . . . I wouldn't seek out that person as my doctor. I want someone I run into at the supermarket." Moreover, several patients stress that in a small town physicians would have virtually no social life if they avoided friendships with their patients. When asked whether they would prefer to see a physician with whom they did not have a social relationship, the answer was unanimous: all nine patients chose to stay with their physician/friend.

One concern with dual relationships, shared by both patients and physicians, was a potential loss of objectivity in the professional relationship. Interestingly, patients tended to see this as an advantage; physicians, as a disadvantage. Patients perceived that their physicians would be more personally involved in their care. One patient cited an example of a visit to an orthopedic surgeon in Portland several years ago. He was able to see the surgeon only after several months of waiting, at which time the surgeon recommended physical therapy. "I felt like a number," he grumbled. Returning to this small town, he called an orthopedic surgeon with whom he fished regularly and was operated on within the week. "I had a better outcome when I was treated by a friend." Another pointed out, "When you want things done in the world, you call a friend . . . your friend the banker, your friend the lawyer. Or your friend the doctor."

Physicians, however, worried that this loss of objectivity could compromise their ability to assess the patient meticulously. "One is blind to the things he doesn't want to see. . . . You think, that couldn't happen to my friend." One physician emphasized that, though he enjoyed many dual relationships, he was cautious to refer a patient if he felt he was "too close to see the whole picture."

Similar to the patients, physicians found the close relationship to be both beneficial and detrimental. They identified a "very positive interaction" that could foster the growth of both the personal and professional relationship. Many physicians stated that they would evaluate a friend on a "case-by-case basis" to determine if they could care for him or her as a patient. Altogether, physicians demonstrated that the priority lies first and foremost with the patient. They were willing to accommodate their patient's wishes, and to refer him or her if so desired. One physician aptly stated, "You must treat a friend as you would anyone else. You discuss the alternatives and the risks, and you allow them to make the decision that is best for them."

Physicians generally found that dual relationships were extremely difficult, even impossible, to avoid in a small town. Many made attempts to avoid them; others embraced them. Yet all agreed that remaining objective was essential to maintaining professionalism. "You have to follow the standard of care as you would with any patient. If it's a friend, you have to be extra conscious. Keep asking yourself, am I doing enough here? Am I doing more than I would for anyone else?"

I was faced with my first dual relationship in the emergency department that day. Alternating between comforting the nurse, with whom I worked regularly in the hospital, and caring for her grandfather, I was apprehensive of whether my close proximity would color my ability to care objectively. It did not. Instead, I was honored to care for this nurse and her grandfather in their time of need. I witnessed firsthand the frank honesty and communication exchanged between the family and their physician. I saw an unspoken understanding that comes only from years of friendship.

During my rural rotation, I discovered a new side of medicine. I witnessed physicians who hunt and fish with their patients, patients who curbside their physicians for medical advice in the grocery store. Lawyers who work for their physicians, and physicians who work for their barbers. Relationships that may challenge the sterile guidelines made by medical associations but are nonetheless fruitful. So fruitful in fact, that patients praise their physicians with a loyalty that has become rare in medicine. I am the fourth generation in a line of family practitioners. Over a century of medicine, my family's practice has migrated from the rural farmland of my great-grandfather's practice to that of my father's in a medium-sized metropolitan city. My grandfather's seasoned leather doctor's bag sits in our living room, now only an heirloom, reminiscent of a passed time. A time of house calls, of physicians who care for generations of families. In many rural communities, that era continues to flourish.

And no ethical recommendation can change that.

Published in *Journal of the American Medical Association* 297.4 (2007): 343–44.

Mississippi Mayhem
Hinds County, MS, 2001

C. D. BRADLEY-JENNETT

"Remember you're just an observer"
The ID doctor with the long gray hair and tortoise shell rimmed glasses reminds
    me
I don't need reminding.
I know this is her clinic
I know she is trying to help
I am just an observer here
I am just a resident
Just a witness

Jesse James is black
Really beautiful
Dark like mahogany
Cheek bones angled just so . . . like a model really
But he is dying
"Got that AIDS," he says, matter of factly
He is 26
The medicines might've worked if he'd taken them right
Not "every now and then" as his mother divulges

Now he sits on the examining table, bones jutting out everywhere
"What hurts you?" the doctor says
"Everything," he replies
"And I just keep runnin' to the bathroom . . .
Won't stop no matter what I do . . ."

"Jesse, we need to think about hospice"
"Remember we talked about that . . ."
"I'm having a hard time remembering anything lately. Mrs. . . . I mean Dr. Lee . . .
just tell my mama . . . she remembers everything"

And she does . . . the positive test . . . pregnancy test . . . 27 years ago . . . how
   they had to "remove her womb and everything else" because she wouldn't
   stop bleeding . . . ensuring Jesse would be an
   only child.
She remembered everything . . . the first step, the first word, the first day of
   school . . . the first clue . . . that something just wasn't right . . .
he was 19 and losing weight and kept getting rashes on his face that just looked
   funny and then pneumonia and almost dying like that in Jackson Memorial
   Hospital . . .
They drove 40 miles to get there . . . he needed to see the specialist. She needed
   her baby to live.
The other positive test . . .
"Yes, it was for sure."
"No, they couldn't tell how long he had it."
"Maybe she should talk to him about it."

She had warned him about so much:
"Be careful crossing Fitzgerald road 'less you get hit by a tractor or somethin'"
"Don't swim in Hinds county creek, the waters too dirty, bound to get all kinds
   of germs . . ."
"Pleeeeze, don't get that fast girl pregnant now . . . you know I don't need a baby
   around here . . . with me working all day"
"Baby, I know it's the 20th century, but please don't sass them white folks . . .
   Mississippi ain't changed that much"

Hadn't warned him about this. This disease that would kill him.
He was disappearing right before her eyes.
Shrinking . . . folding in upon himself.
Graying . . . his skin and even patchy areas of his once thick and lush hair.
She remembered everything, but she kept quiet.
And even after she lost her only child, she found it hard to say it aloud.
Everyone knew what Dr. Lee's clinic was for, but it was still a secret in this small
Mississippi town where separate and unequal still reigned supreme.
And everyone said, "Mrs. James, I'm so sorry about your loss," and the deacon-
   esses from the church baked cakes and the supervisor from her job made her
   famous deviled eggs and the pastor's wife fried chicken and people whispered
   laughter . . . as was appropriate for a repast, and everyone was so polite . . .
But, I wanted to shout because Jesse was younger than me and quite possibly
   brighter than me . . .
and now he was dead and that was not OK with me . . .

And I wanted to scream . . . and I wanted to sound the alarm . . . and I wanted
    to rally . . . and I wanted to educate about how it's done up North
. . . but mostly I wanted to scream . . .
but I was just an observer.

If You Don't Have What You Want

JOSEPH GIBES

I drove along in the bright sunshine, counting farmhouses. Third farm on the left—there it was. A few inches of snow lay on the ground, and the lane to the farmhouse was unplowed. As I turned in, I tried to drive in the tracks left by previous vehicles. These were not the marks left by a car or tractor, but the smooth tracks left by wagon or carriage wheels. This was an Amish farm, home of Elim King.

The Amish population in the rural Wisconsin county where I practiced family medicine had grown from nothing, when I started practice, to a substantial community. They generally delivered their babies at home but would bring the baby boys in to our small hospital to be circumcised. For convenience and to avoid incurring the facility charge associated with using the outpatient department, they had approached me about doing home circumcisions. After some discussion with the hospital and the other local docs, I thought it would be a good service to provide and agreed to give it a try. Today was my first one.

As I drove into the yard, I noticed two or three little faces, shy but curious, looking at me through the partially open barn door. I waved at them; they smiled nervously and disappeared. I took my bag from the car seat beside me. The hospital had provided all of the instruments for the procedure, and the nurse and I had gone over all of it before I set out, making sure that everything was there: the clamps and probe, gauze, the drape, the restraint board that helped to immobilize the child during the procedure; and the Mogen clamp, the instrument used to ensure that during the removal of the infant's foreskin, a more radical amputation was not inadvertently performed. I would be out in a remote part of the county with no hope of retrieving a forgotten item.

I had made many home visits to farms before, but I felt strangely out of place as I walked up to the door. There was still a doorbell button on the wall, apparently left over from the previous owners; the Amish do not use electricity. I knocked. No answer. I was about half an hour later than the time I had said I would arrive. Hoping that the farmer hadn't given up on me and headed out to the barn, I knocked again.

This time the door opened, and there stood Mr. King, tall, balding, with the usual beard worn by all of the married men in their community, and the standard black attire. His face lighted up when he saw me. "Hello, Gibes," he said. (Many of my Amish patients just called me by my last name rather than "doctor.")

"Hello, Mr. King. Sorry if I'm a bit late. I was stuck at the clinic by—"

"No problem." I got the impression that the tyrannical rule of the clock did not extend to this farm. "And just call me Elim." He ushered me into a large room that served as the kitchen, dining room, and living room. It was quite warm, heated by a large stove in one corner.

I had been to this farm before, and I remembered that there had been several smaller rooms where there was now one large room. "You've made some changes," I observed.

"Aye, we widened it out a bit to make room for the church." The Amish have no church buildings; rather, they meet in each other's homes.

There were several children playing quietly on one side of the room. Elim said something to them in the Dutch dialect they use, and they quickly collected their playthings and disappeared.

His wife Rebekah came out of a back room. When she saw me, she greeted me warmly. "Well, hello, doctor! How are you doing?"

"Fine, thanks. How are you and the little one?"

"Oh, doing great, thanks. Here, come in and see him." I followed her into the dimly lit bedroom, where the little boy—as yet unnamed—lay in a bassinet. Elim followed us and looked with evident pride at his son.

"That's a good-looking boy you've got there," I said. "What a blessing!"

"Yes, they are, aren't they?" Elim said quietly. Something in his voice caught my attention, and I looked at him closely; even in the dim light I could see his eyes welling up. I was surprised by this thirty-something-year-old farmer, looking at his twelfth child as if he were his first and only one. "No matter how many we have, each one's a little miracle," he said.

We stood there gazing on the miracle for a few moments. Then Rebekah said, "Well, I'd better let you get to work," and she excused herself.

"Will this be enough light for you?" asked Elim. It was quite dark, with heavy curtains over the window; but my eyes had grown accustomed to the light, and I said I thought it would be no problem. I proceeded to unpack the kit and lay out the contents on the neatly made bed. I tabulated everything in my mind as I made a little sterile field and laid the instruments out on it. I was sure everything was there.

"Are you sure you want to watch this, Elim?"

"Oh sure, I've seen plenty before." Four of his children were sons, so I supposed he had.

I gently lifted the little patient from the bassinet and laid him on the board, molded to cradle a newborn baby, and secured his legs with the Velcro straps. He struggled and fussed for a few seconds, but then settled back down, oblivious to his fate.

I put on the gloves and started the procedure. Elim gently held a pacifier with a little sugar water on its tip in his son's mouth, which was enough to keep him quiet. I tried to keep up a little conversation with the farmer as I worked. "Cold, isn't it?"

"Yes," he replied. "I think it gets even colder here than it did in Pennsylvania."

"What kind of stove is that you have?"

"Kerosene."

While we spoke I worked quickly. Two clamps on. Probe to reduce adhesions. Third clamp on, to mark the extent of the foreskin to be removed. Then apply the Mogen clamp and close it. The patient remained stoically quiet through the whole thing. The procedure was all over except for the actual cutting.

I reached to the sterile field for the scalpel. I couldn't see it in the dim light. I pushed the instruments around, looked under the gauze: no scalpel. Trying to sound calm, I asked Elim, "Is there anything else in the kit?"

The farmer obliged by reaching in and feeling around. "Nope," he said.

It suddenly seemed to be getting warmer in the little room, and I started to sweat. The nurse and I had checked and double-checked, and I had checked again, to be sure that everything was there, and we had missed the most important instrument.

The scalpel.

It was a twenty-five minute drive from the clinic and hospital. A little apologetically, I asked the farmer, "Do you have any kind of knife I could borrow?"

If he thought this a strange request, his face did not betray it. He stepped out of the room and said something in their own language to Rebekah. A moment later he returned, bearing in his hand the instrument his wife had found, an eight-inch steak knife. "Will this do?"

Given the situation, I wasn't sure I was going to get anything better. Fortunately, this part of the procedure required neither a sterile instrument nor finesse. "Sure," I said, trying to sound nonchalant, trying to sound as if doing a circumcision with an eight-inch steak knife was a routine occurrence.

The knife was quite dull, and I had to saw at it a bit to get the job done. The patient lay there placidly, Elim looked on placidly, and I tried to look placid. I left the clamp on for another minute and a half to minimize any bleeding. When I removed the clamp, there he was, as good as if I had used the finest sterile precision surgical instrument in the world.

I put a petrolatum gauze dressing on the surgical site and replaced the diaper.

I felt hot and very uncomfortable, and could tell I was blushing; fortunately, in the dim light, the farmer didn't seem to notice. "Well, thank you, Gibes," he said, as I handed his son back to him.

I cleaned up the makeshift operating table and gave some instructions for the care of the surgical wound. We walked out into the large room. It seemed very bright after the dark bedroom. Rebekah came over. "How'd he do?"

"He did great," Elim replied. I wasn't sure if he was referring to his son or me.

"Well, thank you so much, doctor," she said. "We sure appreciate you coming out. Would you like something to eat?"

"No, no thanks, I'd best be getting back."

"All right, Gibes," said Elim. He retrieved a checkbook and wrote out a check for the amount we had agreed on. He and Rebekah thanked me, profusely, again. We shook hands, and I made my way out the door.

Once outside, I started to berate myself in earnest. *I can't BELIEVE I was so stupid to forget a scalpel! They must think I'm an idiot!* Nevertheless, I attempted to keep up an air of nonchalance as I walked to my car. I opened the door and collapsed into the seat. The mental strain of maintaining a matter-of-fact exterior and trying not to appear completely inept had exhausted me.

I sat and stared out the window for a moment, and as I did, in the midst of my self-reproach, a phrase suddenly popped into my head, a phrase I had heard from a missionary doctor while I was a resident working in a bush hospital in Kenya: "If you don't have what you want, you gotta want what you have."

Well, that certainly was true in this situation. And as I stopped berating myself long enough to realize what had just happened, I started to smile. I couldn't help it, as I thought about it: the absurdity of the situation, the complete stupidity in forgetting the scalpel, me sawing away with a kitchen utensil; and the farmer and his wife so gracious and thankful. The smile became a good belly laugh, and I laughed and laughed until tears rolled down my cheeks.

I was still laughing as I drove down the long driveway. *Only in rural practice!* I thought how I was going to tell everyone back in my own world about the day's events:

"Y' know, I'm probably the only doctor in the world to perform a circumcision with an eight-inch steak knife. . . ."

Mom and Pop Doc Shop

DEBORAH LEE LUSKIN

For sixteen years, I managed my husband's medical practice. I called it the Mom and Pop Doc Shop because it was as antiquated as an old-time general store, one where the proprietors lived in back and knew who would come in when, what they would buy, and when they would pay, if ever. Our office was never so quaint as to be attached to our house, but that never stopped patients from dropping by after hours for an informal consultation. And like a store, it took both of us to run it.

Tim and I met in 1984, the year he arrived in Townshend as a doctor for the National Health Service Corps, which had paid his Dartmouth Medical School tuition in return for three years' work. When the three years were up, Tim and I were already married, and the practice became ours—lock, stock, and receivables. The only problem: Tim was too busy doctoring to take care of the books. I, however, had just completed my doctorate in English literature and was unemployed and pregnant. We consulted a business adviser, opened a checking account with two thousand dollars, and on July 1, 1987, we opened for business.

To Tim's patients, the change was seamless. The office location and phone number remained the same, as did the staff. What changed was our need to make a profit, since the National Health Service Corps was no longer footing the bill. After paying our employees' wages and benefits, after paying the rent and utilities, and after buying the Band-Aids and injectibles, we still needed to have money left over to pay ourselves. For sixteen years, and sometimes by the skin of our teeth, we succeeded. And then, on July 1, 2003, we gave the practice away to the local hospital.

Again, to Tim's patients, the change was seamless. The biggest changes were a regular paycheck with generous benefits for Tim and freedom from health care management for me. While there had been significant changes in medical practice during those years, the biggest changes were administrative, including debilitating governmental regulations and the health insurance industry's takeover of the delivery of primary care, changes that introduced excesses of paperwork and a reduction in payments that made staying independent and profitable ever more difficult. Two other factors also contributed to closing the store. One, ironically, was the cost of providing health insurance for our employees and ourselves. The other was the intangible cost to our family.

When Tim first arrived in Townshend, he was one of two family physicians covering the emergency room at Grace Cottage Hospital, a nineteen-bed outpost thirty minutes from Brattleboro Memorial Hospital and an hour and a half from Hanover, where the Mary Hitchcock Hospital was then located. When he asked me to marry him, I said, "Yes—but I'll wait until there's a third doctor in town." Miraculously, the third doctor materialized the following year; for eight years, it was the three of them sharing call. In addition to being the doc on call, Tim also took and developed whatever X-rays he needed, drew blood and ran labs, went on ambulance calls, and served as regional medical examiner. Everything took time, time away from his clinical practice, which is what generated our income.

Back then, interventionist cardiology was still a dream, and bypass surgery was reserved for only the toughest cases. Before the widespread use of statins to treat hyperlipidemia and clot-busting drugs to interrupt myocardial infarctions, heart attacks (as they used to be called) were a common occurrence. Little could be done besides wait one out and then transport the patient to Brattleboro or Dartmouth. In those days, the ambulance service was a volunteer affair (the ambulance itself a retired hearse), and Tim often rode in back, offering what care he could on the trip up and catching whatever shut-eye he could in the empty gurney on the return.

In 1987 few of Tim's patients had health insurance. Those who did were in-sured against calamity; they carried major medical policies that covered injury and illness after meeting an annual deductible. Charges for the family doctor's care of injury or illness could be applied to that deductible, but charges for rou-tine wellness care could not. Annual physicals and well-child visits typically had to be paid for out of pocket, setting patients back about seventeen-dollars.

From a business point of view, the bookkeeping was fairly simple. As patients left the office they paid their bills and were given receipts to send to their insurance companies for reimbursement. Except for Blue Cross Blue Shield, Medicare, and Medicaid, our office did not usually interfere in the patient-insurer relationship; we only provided the health care. It is this that has dramatically changed.

We had inherited aging receivables with the practice, purchased one of the few medical software programs on the market, and became the first computer users in the local medical community. Computerization proved so much more efficient than our manual system that we began billing on behalf of our patients. Before long, we became the middlemen, running between insurer and subscriber, trying to get paid.

At first, our business prospered and our family flourished. We quickly had three healthy children and, between the two of us, were earning a comfortable salary by local, if not medical, standards. My job at the office was part time; Tim worked twelve- to fourteen-hour days, and he covered the emergency room at Grace Cottage Hospital every third night. He also delivered babies. There were days when he didn't see his own. He yearned for family time; I craved his companionship and partnership in parenting.

Our children would ask, "Is Dad on call?" the nights Tim didn't return by bedtime. If we hadn't seen him in a few days, we'd visit him at the hospital and join him for a meal or stop by his office and raid the pediatric drawer for stickers. Tim wanted to be with his children and would rush home to give baths when he could. After stories, songs, and "goodnight," he'd return to the office to finish his charts. In 1990 we'd bought and renovated a building for the growing practice, incurring our first large debt. Three years after moving in, Tim was working harder with less family time, and our income had plunged. Yes, we were building equity, but equity doesn't buy milk at the store.

My father, a successful businessman, had counseled us that there were only three ways to increase profit: cut costs, increase productivity, and raise prices. We'd done the first two, and, in the highly regulated health care industry, there were strict limits to what we could do about the third. Medicare and Medicaid accounted for half of Tim's practice—or "payor mix," in the lingo of the jargon-laden industry. Medicare and Medicaid are government-issued insurance, and in the pay-for-service model, the government first sets the price it will pay, and then it takes a 20 percent discount. In my most exhausted and somewhat bitter days, I proposed that after we figured our federal tax liability, we only send in 80 percent. Just the idea cheered me up.

There was a way to improve our Medicare and Medicaid reimbursement—if we were willing to take on the added work of becoming a Rural Health Clinic (RHC). The Rural Health Clinic program was established in 1977 to address an inadequate supply of physicians who serve Medicare and Medicaid beneficiaries in rural areas. Like the National Health Service, which brings physicians to medically underserved areas, Rural Health Clinics aim to keep them there. The paperwork alone could anchor a practice in place. After considering our options—most of which included packing up and moving—we hired consultants, borrowed money to pay them, and applied.

Over time, we learned how to fulfill the often redundant, sometimes opaque, reporting requirements of being an RHC. We had to have written job descriptions: I was now practice manager, head of human resources, director of information technology, director of facilities, and safety officer. I had to conduct annual fire drills—*and document them.* We also learned that while we had strict deadlines to meet with our reports—complete with interest and penalties—Medicare and Medicaid could take forever to audit our reports. Nevertheless, for several years we were able to pay our bills, pay an office cleaner, pay ourselves, raise wages, and fund a profit-sharing plan for retirement.

Physicians sometimes stumbled across Grace Cottage when they were vacationing in southern Vermont; others heard about this tiny hospital through some medical grapevine. Whenever a doctor expressed interest in setting up shop, we'd have them for dinner, one couple trying to seduce another to join in what was unquestionably a good life that would be so much better if there was one more doc with whom to share call.

It was how Tim practiced medicine that was so appealing, not his income. He was his own boss; he treated whole families; he made house calls; he was part of the social fabric of the town in which he served. Other bonuses included a two-mile commute and casual dress every day of the week. Our small-town life was bucolic: we grew lots of vegetables, tended a flock of chickens, kept bees, and even raised our own pig. We lived smack in the midst of New England's beauty and could snowshoe out our back door or head into the Green Mountain National Forest within minutes.

After ten years of being on call every third night, a fourth doctor came to town. Unlike the three other family practitioners in town, however, this physician was hired by the hospital. Once there were four docs in the call schedule and a guaranteed living wage, working in Townshend became more attractive. Shortly thereafter, the hospital hired a fifth doctor, then a sixth. At one time recently, the call schedule included seven physicians, but it didn't last.

Meanwhile, managed care arrived, adding a huge, unreimbursed workload to our practice. Different companies and different policies covered different services. Staff researched patients' policies to find out what a patient's coverage would allow Tim to do. Instead of Tim providing the care his patients required, he was providing the care the patients' insurers allowed. We submitted claims on behalf of our patients in order to be paid by their insurers. We were blessed with employees who worked hard for our patients, who were loyal to Tim, and who were forgiving of me.

In the early years, I resented our employees' annual raises. As we worked together, however, I came to appreciate these women, wished I could pay them more, and considered them our allies. Nevertheless, the economic reality was that their hourly wage was about half the cost of their employment. Wages triggered taxes for social security, Medicare, workman's compensation, unemployment, six paid holidays, and two to three weeks paid vacation. We also offered nontaxable benefits, such as paid lunches, profit sharing, and health insurance.

Too often, our employees chose to forgo raises in return for paid health insurance premiums, which rose yearly. To stay ahead of the curve, we kept switching to policies with higher co-pays and higher deductibles; the business picked up employees' out-of-pocket costs after the first two hundred dollars. In our penultimate year in business, three employees met our $2,500 deductible. It was a very lean year.

It was also a year of staff illness and absence from work. In addition to my management duties, I was now filling in where ever I could. Some patients loved when I answered the phone and they could chat with the doctor's wife; others, understandably, didn't want me involved in their care. I didn't want to be there.

When we married, Tim and I made a pact not to stifle each other. With the kids in school and despite the demands of the medical practice, I had managed to draft two novels, publish articles, and teach on a limited basis. Those were the things I was uniquely good at; I was not as good at answering the phone, and posting payments only heightened my awareness of how fragile our finances were becoming again.

But it wasn't just a matter of finances. We probably could have accepted the grim realities of diminishing income, unpaid vacations, inadequate retirement savings, and expensive health insurance if it weren't for two things: summers and HIPAA.

Summers were always difficult. The kids, home from school, needed us. Even if we could have afforded summer-long camps, we didn't want to send our kids away. While the problem of finding good summertime childcare is not unique to medical families, the unpredictability of Tim's availability created both a challenge and a tension, leaving the logistics and transportation to me. In order for me to manage the office, we enrolled the kids in local day camps, creating a daily logistical challenge of playdates and carpools. With good weather, Tim and I also wanted to get out and play, have family time, or at least get ahead of the weeds in the garden. But summer brought with it a significant number of visitors hell-bent on having a good time, often landing them in the ER. Not only was the ER busier in summer, but the on-call rotation was accelerated, as at least one doctor each week was away on vacation.

The summer of 2002 was the worst. We had taken our three kids on a service mission, where we helped run a drama and arts camp for orphans in Russia. It was a three-week trip, the longest we'd ever been away from the office. When we returned, it took another three weeks to recover, but a snafu in the call schedule had Tim on call six days out of twelve. August, easily the busiest month in the ER, was made busier the evening Tim was admitted.

Tim wanted to check the bees we'd neglected most of the summer. It was too hot and sticky, I told him. Not good bee weather. I went for a walk. Tim looked in on the bees by himself. Despite his suit and helmet, the bees mobbed him, triggering anaphylaxis. By the time I returned, Tim had already injected himself with epinephrine. He gave himself a second injection as I drove him to Grace Cottage, where he was treated. The next morning, he was back at work and on call.

With the bees back in the hive and the children back in school, I faced the task of trying to understand the Health Insurance Portability and Accountability Act, better known as HIPAA. We had already weathered CLIA (Clinical Laboratory Improvement Amendments), which standardized the lab, and EMTALA (Emergency Medical Treatment and Active Labor Act), the hospital anti-dumping law. HIPAA was initially passed in 1996, but its Privacy Rule was scheduled to go into effect in April 2003. It was not clear to me if or how the law would protect our patients' privacy more or even any differently from how we already guarded their personal health information. It was clear that this meant yet more paperwork for our staff and another added expense. An eleventh-hour reprieve for small entities allowed us an added year before we had to have all our forms in place. I didn't see how another year would make any significant difference to the bottom line. Complying with HIPAA would have required us to retool our information technology yet again. It would hold us individually and collectively accountable for noncompliance, including fines and criminal charges. Who was writing these laws?

People in Washington were writing these laws. In the winter and spring of 2003, I talked with people at both the state and federal levels about turning our little RHC into a Federally Qualified Health Center, the hub in a network stretching across at least two counties in Southern Vermont. It was a huge undertaking, thrilling and scary and much more interesting than trying to figure out how to implement HIPAA. I purchased a power suit from the local thrift shop, which I wore to a few meetings. It just didn't fit. I didn't really want to be a health care administrator, nor could Tim or I see how we could support ourselves through the transition. So, I made one more attempt to understand HIPAA. I'm trained to read closely, to see both text and subtext. The Privacy Rule presents itself as a means of protecting sensitive health information, but what it really does is grant government, law enforcement, and insurance companies access to personal health records. This was not a game I wanted to play. Instead of putting HIPAA into place, we entered negotiations with Grace Cottage Hospital to take over our practice. At the end of the day on June 30, we closed up shop.

It was hardest on our employees. Even though the hospital matched their wages, offered them more and better benefits, and transferred their years of service, they were used to working for us, and that changed. As one former employee recently told me, "It was like a family. Our patients were like family. Our coworkers were like family. I really miss it." Over the years, this woman served as receptionist, bookkeeper, substitute office nurse, insurance coder, and bill collector—sometimes all in the same day. Now, she's a certified medical billing specialist, and that's all she does, in her isolated cubicle, every working day.

To my surprise, I sometimes miss it too. I don't miss our Wednesday night pillow talk, which was always about whether we'd make Thursday's payroll; I don't miss the cost reports; I prefer not knowing who owes money for care. But I do miss my former staff and our teamwork—how we all pulled together to provide excellent, personalized care for our patients, and for each other. I've moved on, however, developing a growing practice as a freelance teacher, researcher and writer, often writing about physicians and medicine.

For Tim, what has changed is a regular paycheck and freedom to practice medicine without the headaches of running a business as well. Otherwise, much remains the same. Despite paid personal days and sick leave, he has yet to use one. He is still on call too often, is late for dinner more often than not, and invariably works several hours on his days off. Since signing on with Grace Cottage, he has been named Medical Director, and he spends countless hours in meetings as well.

What has not changed is that Tim is still there, doing what he does best: giving patients his whole attention, providing the kind of primary care that takes good listening skills, sharp observation, knowledge of both a patient's medical and social history, and the time to give comprehensive care.

A version of this piece was published as "Care Package" in *Dartmouth Medicine*, Fall 2007.

Stopping by Malnati's Meadow

RICHARD M. BERLIN

Stopping by Malnati's meadow I see
he has rolled his hay into huge round bales
ten feet tall, almost eighty scattered near
and far in the late summer sun. A red-tailed
hawk claims one for his perch and waits
for his mate, while overhead a pair of kestrels
flash cinnamon wings against a cobalt sky.
Yesterday, my eighty-year-old mother
tripped and fell over her own two feet, nothing
injured except her spirit, my father dead
almost half my life, my doctor-wife treating
kids on the other side of Lenox Mountain,
me standing here alone like the maple
Malnati left in his meadow, green leaves
catching the sun's September fire.

When Hostility Melted for the "Funny Accent"

GODFREY ONIME

The truth will set you free, but first it will piss you off.
—MAL PANCOAST

I hit the snooze button of my alarm clock several times that Sunday morning before the need to hurry sent me scurrying about like a poisoned rat. I was already at the hospital before realizing I was wearing different colored socks—a light khaki brown and a darker brown. So, whenever I had to sit, I first tugged my pants down to my hips like a teenage boy to hide my socks.

Not that I had much opportunity to sit down, anyway. Every patient and every nurse screamed for my attention. I was in the midst of stabilizing a middle-aged man with pericardial effusion—that is, life threatening fluid around his heart—when my beeper went off—again. When I returned the page, it was the emergency room nurse reminding me about another patient waiting to be admitted.

"The family is getting angry that he's still in the ER," she complained.

I wanted to scream, "Did you tell them I have sicker patients to deal with, plus I've barely had four hours of sleep in the past two days?" But I did not. Instead, I told her to tell the almighty family that I was not simply sitting crossed-legs drinking *Mocha* and calling Geico to save on my car insurance. This was meant as a joke, but the nurse was not amused. I suspect she relayed the message to the family exactly as the doctor ordered.

Another hour later, finally managing to have the patient with the pericardial effusion airlifted to the Duke University Medical Center, a bigger and better-equipped facility than my community hospital in the southeastern region of North Carolina, I dashed to the ER. My new patient, Mr. Common—elderly, frail, taciturn—was sitting propped up on his stretcher and intermittently dozing. An IV line dripped fluids into a delicate vein in his wrinkled forearm. I drew the thick curtain to provide privacy from the rest of the ER, but it was not enough to block the shrieks of an infant the ER physician was attending to a few rooms away.

Mr. Common's family—two sons, a daughter, and a daughter-in-law—had been sitting by his bed. They promptly rose, as if orchestrated, when I entered the room and hovered about the tiny space, crowding me. The somber look on their faces was unnerving—that look that commonly made me stammer as a rookie intern. But internship was almost a decade ago, and I liked to think I had "toughed up" over the years. I apologized for keeping Mr. Common waiting, explaining that it had been a terribly busy day.

"We have been here for over six hours," Elvis, the eldest son complained. He appeared in his early fifties and had flowing blond hair that covered his ears. He had a habit of jerking his head every so often, which kept his hair flying, revealing a diamond earring imbedded in his left earlobe.

"I'm sorry you had such a long wait," I apologized again, "but I only heard about your father some two hours ago." That is one problem many non-ER doctors face when admitting patients to the hospital. When the patients come to the emergency room, they are first evaluated by the ER physicians. Often, tests must be done before the physicians can decide whether to admit or discharge a patient. If the decision is made to admit, only then does the admitting physician hear about it; unfortunately, by then, the patient may have already been in the ER for several hours, and any delay added by the admitting physician gravely compounds the problem. I explained this to the family as best as I could, also apprising them there were other sick patients in the hospital who needed my urgent attention.

"Let's just get admitting him over with," Elvis snapped.

I proceeded to obtain their father's history. His stools had been dark the past week and he had gotten progressively weaker. He had a history of gastrointestinal ulcer, which had ruptured in the past, almost killing him and necessitating surgery. He took a blood pressure medication, another for enlarged prostate, one for stomach acid and, per his doctor's recommendation, an aspirin a day. No, he had never suffered a heart attack or stroke. When I shone my penlight into his eyes, the sclera was so white it matched the sleeve of my lab coat. His skin was pale, even more noticeably so against my dark hands as I pushed on his belly; the abdomen was soft and nontender. I reviewed his labs and saw that his red blood cells, the oxygen-carrying component of his blood, were low.

I decided that Mr. Common had had moderately severe gastrointestinal bleeding and indeed required hospitalization. He would need blood transfusion as well. I further informed the family that I'd have the gastroenterologist see him the following day for evaluation with likely upper endoscopy—a long fiber optic tube with a camera at the tip guided down his throat to look at his stomach and the early part of his small intestine, the duodenum—and, if that was unrevealing for the source of his bleeding, a different but similar tube inserted through his rectum, a procedure called colonoscopy. "I can always be reached if there are problems," I concluded, "but I'll see him again tomorrow."

"What time?" the daughter demanded. About five feet five and slim, she—unlike her brother Elvis but like her father—seemed frugal with words. "We'd like to be present when you see him tomorrow."

I had patients scheduled at the clinic from nine until five the next day, and, so far, eight or nine others on my hospital service. I informed the Commons that baring an emergency, I should see their father between seven and nine o'clock in the morning.

"You mind if I ask where you from?" she asked. "I love the way you talk."

"Nigeria," I told her, my face cringing.

The next day, not daring to press the snooze on my alarm clock and taking extra care to pick matching socks, I arrived at the hospital just after seven. Hoping to allow enough time for all the children to be present, I did not go see Mr. Common first but started the day with an ICU patient—a middle-aged woman with pneumonia who was on the ventilator and barely staying alive. Some forty-five minutes later I was still combing through her case, but I couldn't think of what else to do for her. As I wrote my final orders on her chart, I kept looking at my gold-plated watch, repeating the same gesture as I saw my other ICU patient with alcohol withdrawal. Thankfully, he was doing better and since bed crunch was always a problem at the ICU, I wrote an order to transfer him to a medical but monitored bed.

It was 8:05 A.M. when I got to Mr. Common's room. Only his daughter was present. The gastroenterologist had not been to see the old man yet. After re-examining him, listening to his lungs and chest and palpating his abdomen to make sure it was not tender, I updated the daughter about her father's stable condition. I had also checked his blood count for that morning and further assured her it had improved. Then I tried to leave to go see my other patients before hurrying to the clinic, but she proceeded to ask over and over again the same questions I had just answered.

I was finally leaving Mr. Common's room when Elvis arrived, his wife at his side. "How's Dad doing?" he asked.

"He's stable," I said.

Then Elvis asked the same questions I had answered for his sister. I told him I had to go and suggested that the family talk amongst themselves, but it was like yelling at a radio to stop talking.

No sooner was I finally hunched over Mr. Common's chart at the nurse's station, scribbling my notes, when the patient representative called me aside. "Mr. Common is your patient, right?" she asked.

"Is there a problem?" I retorted, somewhat on the defensive.

"The son complained that they were kept waiting for too long at the ER yesterday."

My face grew hot in spite of the central air conditioning. I loosened my tie, but my throat was too dry to make any sound, plus I'd learned to keep quiet when I felt rage.

"I understand it was very busy over the weekend," the rep continued, "but you know we have to follow up on these complaints. And I'm supposed to remind you about the hospital's mission that you make every effort to see a patient within half an hour of receiving the call from the ER."

"Thanks," I said. "Now that you've done your job, I better go continue with mine before I get fired by the hospital."

"You know it's not like that," the rep was saying, but the increased blood flow from my galloping heart made me strong and I left her in mid-sentence.

How dare the Commons or, more specifically, that Elvis guy! What did they expect the hospital to do with me, anyway? Take away my license? I always knew they did not like me. Maybe they were racists. Maybe they thought their father was too good to be cared for by a black man, one with an accent that was neither American nor British for that matter. Yes, one patient once accused me, after I refused to prescribe antibiotics for what I suspected a viral upper respiratory infection, of being an African who still believed in the healing powers of rocks and trees and the voodoo dance. I had not even asked to care for their father, for heaven's sake. I'd been on call and their family doctor did not admit patients.

The rest of Mr. Common's hospital stay was as uneventful as I could scheme. I just wanted to take good care of my patients, not fight with family members. I alternated rounding very early in the morning with late in the day to avoid his children, but I always called to update them on his condition. It was a pity they kept missing me, they said; I expressed my disappointments too.

One day I found the old man on his back in bed, eyes closed, breaths regular. His upper body was exposed in the chilly room. Not wanting to disturb his sleep, I pulled the blanket over his gray-haired chest. Then I began to sneak out of the room.

"Doctor?" The old man called, almost in a whisper.

I turned to see what he wanted.

"Thank you," he said.

It did not escape me that these were probably the only words I'd heard him utter without repeated prompting. "You're quite welcome," I replied.

The gastroenterologist did an upper and lower endoscopy on Mr. Common during that hospitalization and found no significant cause for his bleeding. He suspected it was a self-limiting hemorrhage and placed the patient on iron supplements. When some five days after admission it was time to discharge him, I wished the old man and his family well and instructed them to follow up with his family doctor.

"Thank God," I breathed, after I'd discharged him. That night I celebrated the occasion with a large Mocha at my local Barnes and Noble.

But I was not that lucky, nor was Mr. Common. He returned to the ER just under a month later with further significant anemia. One of my hospital's many policies was that patients needing hospital readmission within thirty days of a discharge returned to the physician who previously cared for them, presumably to enhance continuity of care. It was about 1:00 A.M. when the ER physician called me this time.

Like most community hospitals in America, mine lacked interns and residents. The attending physicians could give the nurses orders by phone and delay seeing patients. But I did no such thing after learning of the case. I was terrified not to go see him now.

Terrified, of course, of his children.

I staggered out of bed and roused myself with cold tap water on my face. As my SUV tore through the deserted road to the hospital, I recalled with dissatisfaction that I was still fighting with the patient's insurance company concerning the bill for his previous hospitalization. Maybe I should join the growing flock of primary care doctors giving up hospital work.

At the ER, the perpetual bright lights gave the illusion of daytime. All three children were present—the two sons and daughter.

Elvis thanked me for responding so promptly. Far from how I felt myself, he stated that they were glad I was the one on call. His father did not like doctors, he said; he agreed to return to the ER only if "the doctor with the funny accent" saw him. I laughed in spite of myself, but after tucking the old man into his hospital bed, making sure to order two units of blood transfusions and another consultation with the gastroenterologist, I was glad to escape back home and delighted to crawl into bed in the hopes of catching a couple of hours of snooze before I had to begin the new day.

The gastroenterologist did not think Mr. Common needed repeat endoscopy but suggested a "capsule" endoscopy, in which the patient swallows a tiny camera that passes through the system so its images can be analyzed.

Again the old man was ready to return home and follow up with his primary care doctor. He was already dressed and sitting up in bed when I arrived at his room. I stared in disbelief when I noted his feet; he wore two different colored socks, a black one on one foot and a green on the other.

"He's in a hurry to go home," his daughter explained. Then, realizing I was not just starring at her dad but at his socks, she added, "His vision is not so good anymore, but he wouldn't change his socks when we told him about it."

Elvis cleared his throat and addressed me. "We've been impressed with the way you cared for Dad," he began. I whirled to face him, not sure I heard him right. He continued: "We have discussed it and we think you should be his primary-care doctor." He jerked his head, hair flying and earring sparkling. "He likes you, plus you also do hospital work. Are you accepting new patients?"

I looked from the children to the old man and back at the children, not sure how to respond. They'd discussed this with each other! Did they make a list of the pros and cons of choosing me as their father's new doctor, hotly debate each point, possibly open to a veto by Elvis? Was I now supposed to ignore their wariness and hostility a month earlier, forget their complaint against me? Or maybe they expected me to hop up and down that they were choosing me, sing joy-oh-joy, dance the voodoo dance.

Then I cautioned myself. Doctors, if not careful, can project their frustration onto their patients. I wondered: Could that be happening here? What wrong had this family done? Weren't families supposed to be advocates of their sick loved ones, demand expedient and optimum care? I realized I was afraid they would discover that at times I could be wrong too.

There was an awkward pause while I thought this out. But really, there was just one answer. "I'll be happy to be his doctor," I said.

A shorter version of this piece was published in the *New York Times* on 27 May 2008.

Mashkikiwinini: Thanking Sylvester for His Unconditional Smile

ARNE VAINIO

It wasn't easy becoming a physician. But I didn't do it by myself. I've had help and guidance all along from well-educated people and teachers who spent their lives helping others advance. I've had lots of great teachers and would like to publicly thank them but was told I may not be able to use names without written permission and a release form. This may complicate things, but I'll get it done somehow.

Sometimes teaching comes when you aren't looking for it or even have the time to think about it. Recently, one of my partners at Min-No-Aya-Win Human Services Clinic on the Fond du Lac Ojibwe Reservation in Cloquet, Minnesota, was off, and I saw one of her patients. Behind and rushed (as usual), I went over Sylvester's records enough to know he had metastatic cancer, but his records were sketchy and I didn't know much beyond that. Before I went in, one of the nurses commented that she thought he was in denial about his prognosis. That's the expectation I had as I walked into Sylvester's room and introduced myself. I expected to see a man desperately holding out for a cure and a miracle. Instead, I met a smiling man who welcomed me into the room. His eyes were bright and clear, his smile sincere and real. In spite of that, he was pale, gaunt, and clearly sick. He had dark circles under his eyes and his words came in short, labored sentences. His belly was huge, even under his baggy shirt. He was short of breath just sitting on the exam table.

"I would like to know if my cancer is worse. Last year I was told I had five months to live. This year I'm going to plant tomatoes." He had no illusions about his cancer and his prognosis; he knew this was a bad cancer and was spreading.

In the room, I went through his records again and found a CT scan report from six months earlier from a different medical system. The report stated "interval worsening" since his last study, with spread of cancer to multiple areas of his liver, into his abdominal wall muscles, and into the mesenteric area. His cancer was a GIST (gastrointestinal stromal tumor), which is a rare cancer. It can either be slow growing or aggressive. Unfortunately, his was very bad and spreading rapidly. The fact that he had already asked not to be resuscitated was in his records. There wasn't much to do at this point except to make sure he was comfortable and didn't suffer.

On exam his lungs sounded clear in the upper portions but decreased in the lower right side. He lifted his shirt and I could see the massive tumor under the skin on the entire right side of his belly. It was tented up at an unnatural angle and as hard as wood. As I felt around the edges of the tumor, I could feel that it went deep inside his abdomen and I could feel other smaller tumors.

Sometimes diseases that involve the liver cause ascites, fluid collecting inside the abdominal cavity. I could not identify this on exam but was hoping for it, as draining it could help his breathing. A chest X-ray showed part of one of his ribs eaten away and a mass inside his chest. He accepted this without complaint. Through all of this, he was smiling and planning his garden.

Sylvester was accompanied by a social worker. I asked, "Is he always like this?"

"Short of breath?"

"No. Is he always this positive?"

"Always."

I knew as soon as I met him that Sylvester had a gift. Not many could look death in the eye with his grace and dignity. I asked him if he would consent to go to the medical school with me if I could set up a day so medical students could meet him and learn from him. Not just from a cancer standpoint but from a spiritual standpoint and a lesson in the beauty of life.

We can all learn that lesson.

He agreed immediately.

The following week was spring break at the medical school in Duluth where I trained. The week after that, the medical students had preceptorships and were going to be staying with doctors in rural communities. The earliest time to get him to the medical school was three weeks away. I set this up, and he was happy for the opportunity.

Early the next week I got a call from the social worker. Sylvester's breathing was worse. He lived over a hundred miles away and came to our clinic primarily so he could get his free medicines from our pharmacy. Given the distance, getting rides for him was a major complication.

I set up a procedure to try to drain fluid from his belly under ultrasound. Unfortunately, there was no fluid to drain. I then ordered a CT scan of his chest, abdomen, and pelvis to see if the cancer was causing his shortness of breath. His kidney function tests were abnormal and he couldn't tolerate the contrast dye needed for the scan, so he didn't get it. He had gotten up at 4 A.M., rode over two hundred miles, and wasted one of his few precious days.

Later in the week, I got a call from a hospice nurse. Sylvester wasn't necessarily any worse but had finally accepted hospice care to ease his final days.

The next week I got a call from a doctor in the hospital in the town where Sylvester lived. He had been admitted with a fever, but after the workup no source was found. He was becoming increasingly short of breath, confused, and less and less responsive.

I had talked with the social worker the week after my only visit with Sylvester. She told me that on the drive home he was so excited to be going to the medical school. "I'm going to teach doctors! I always worried that I would be forgotten, but now I get to have people remember who I was." She told me that sometimes he would play a harmonica for her in the car. "It was quiet and haunting, sometimes I could barely hear it. It was beautiful."

As I wrote this article, Sylvester was in the hospital and was not expected to survive the night. He was no longer responding, but his family was present. I wanted to be there and to hold his hand, but I was on call and I could not leave. I wanted to thank him for teaching me the beauty of life and making me realize the things we take for granted won't always be there. I wanted to apologize for wasting one of his last days trying to get tests. I wanted to let him know that I'll plant the tomatoes this year. I wanted him to know that he will be remembered.

Always.

He will be some small part of whatever I do from now on. I wanted to say I was sorry for taking so long to get him set up to teach the medical students. His schedule was more important than ours. I wanted to thank him publicly. But I did not have a signed release, but maybe now, I can get his family to allow me the honor.

In Memory of Sylvester LaDuke, February 14, 1942–April 9, 2007

This article appeared in 2007 in News from Indian Country, a national Native American newspaper for which Arne writes a column.

A Psychiatrist Waits for His Ten o'clock Patient and Imagines He Is Han Shan

RICHARD M. BERLIN

Daughter gone,
hair gone, my father
dead for half my life.
Patients I saved from suicide
lived until old age,
died from cancer instead!
Twenty years of hospital work.
Twenty years pruning apple trees
on the west flank of Cold Mountain.
Once they were sticks.
Now the branches bow with ripe fruit.
A faint wind stirs them.
I'll share a bushel with the crows,
another with the worms!

Note: Han Shan was a Taoist/Buddhist hermit-poet who lived in China's Tientai Mountains 1,200 years ago. An immortal figure in Chinese literature and Zen, his name means Cold Mountain, which he used to refer to himself and the mountain retreat where he lived.

Three Days Changed My Grandfather's Life

DAVID MCRAY

My grandfather measured time carefully; dates were important to him. He could proudly recall at least one memory from seventy-six of his seventy-nine years of life, and he could easily remember the exact date on which almost every significant event occurred during his adult years. But three days, spanning across three years, were critical in the story of his life and its final chapter.

In the fall of 1991, his physician had discovered on a routine blood chemistry panel that his creatinine was elevated. The initial investigation was unremarkable, and being a private man, he told his family little. As a result, his discomfort that Christmas was noteworthy. Restless and uncomfortable, he frequently changed positions and quietly scratched his skin. He did not volunteer any information, but when asked, he admitted that he was "freezing and itching." He was certain, however, that his condition did not warrant anyone's concern.

The months following Christmas were filled with additional visits with his physician, referral to larger medical centers, and, finally the kidney biopsy. We talked about his health and the reasons for the various tests and procedures that were being recommended. A young family physician practicing in a small, rural east Tennessee community four hours from his home, I was eager to help. I tried to answer his questions and encouraged him to ask more of his doctors. This was especially difficult for him; he seemed to feel out of place talking with the rapidly expanding collection of physicians who were attending to his case.

A simple, humble man, my grandfather was always aware of his limited education, having only completed the eighth grade. He was concerned that he did not communicate well with learned individuals, and he fretted over the burden he felt he placed on his physicians by his failure to quickly grasp the complexities of his condition. So, coax and encourage as I might, he seldom asked many questions. As a result, I gradually began to serve as his interpreter. He was beginning to understand that he was ill and that his illness would require ongoing management, but he was hopeful, even confident, that his illness could be cured.

The renal biopsy revealed a nonspecific form of glomerulonephritis, untreatable and incurable. Many questions followed: "What did I do wrong? Is it a result of my diet? What should I do now?" My grandfather never understood what was happening to his kidneys—why he continued to urinate without difficulty if his kidneys were "failing," why he became increasingly fatigued, and why he suffered from "low blood" requiring multiple transfusions. I explained what I could, reeducated myself, acknowledged my lack of expertise in this area, but stressed my confidence that his illness was being managed appropriately. Reluctantly, he began to accept that his condition was irreversible, incurable. Yet, all his physicians' attention remained focused on the management of his illness with little attention given to how he was experiencing his illness and the options that might be available to him.

As his creatinine level rose, his hematocrit fell, and by autumn he had no choice. With the itching worse and the fatigue incapacitating, if he wanted to feel better—in fact, if he wanted to continue to live—he needed to begin dialysis. He did not understand what was being offered, how it would work or how it would make him feel. The therapy was never described as a form of life support with all the customary conversations about indications, alternatives, ethics, and options for withdrawal. It was simply the next step in the management of his illness; a step he felt forced to accept but never really did.

On November 1, 1993, the first of the three pivotal dates, his small red ledger, which he had used to carefully track the dates and the cost of his injections and transfusions, contained a very simple and somber entry—"dialysis." From that point on, three times a week, he would make the same entry. The brevity and simplicity of it did not do justice to the effect it had on his life. My grandparents had made their home for over fifty years in the same house in a small town at the foot of a mountain in rural southeast Tennessee. The physician in their community of 1,800 residents had been unable to offer much assistance to my grandparents for many years, so they received their primary medical care from a physician at the regional hospital about fifteen minutes away. The nearest dialysis center was in yet another town, forty-five minutes north. The office of my grandfather's nephrologist was an additional forty-five minutes beyond the center, near the state capital. Three days a week, my grandparents would leave home early in the morning and make the trip to greet the staff and submit to "misery," the word he used to describe the way dialysis made him feel.

Miserable though he was, he made the best of the situation, as he had always done with every hardship he encountered in his life—a two-hour train trip as a child to receive care for a broken arm; an abbreviated education; the Great Depression; the death of premature infants soon after birth in the bedroom of his home; long, rotating shifts as a railroad brakeman; and the accumulated trials and disappointments that compose a life. Even on the bad days, he found the energy and courage to joke with the dialysis nurses. The days he came for his treatment, they later said, were very special days.

For two and a half years, he drove himself to dialysis most of the time. He still traveled some—an occasional trip to visit his children, even a four-hour bus trip to see me. Each journey meant a visit to a different dialysis center—new people and unpredictable experiences.

On April 18, 1996, the second of the three days, a stroke changed everything. He awoke that morning with some troubling weakness and numbness in his right arm and leg. At first he ignored it, but after his symptoms progressed, he agreed to go to the hospital. An ambulance trip and brief evaluation in the local hospital emergency room were followed by a transfer to the major medical center in Nashville where my grandfather remained hospitalized for two weeks. He was discharged to a rehabilitation hospital and then an extended care facility. He never suffered from a severe loss of function, but he became dependent, unable to attend to his most basic needs. His dignity was under attack; his spirit broken. Smiles were less common. Activity was limited to movement from the hospital bed to a chair to the bathroom and back. He said less and moaned more. When asked if he was in pain, he said, "No, I'm in misery. I want to go home."

My grandfather always wanted to go home. Whenever he went anywhere for an extended visit, he soon spoke of needing to go home. Even after retirement, when his obligations at home were less pressing, he felt a "gravitational pull" toward home. While in the hospital and nursing home in Nashville, he was advised to reconsider; the options in the city were better. When he improved, and everyone insisted he would, he would have the choice of other excellent, assisted-living situations. His son lived nearby. Clearly, the best choice was to stay there, but my grandfather insisted on going home. Reluctantly, his family agreed.

Arrangements were made, supplies and equipment purchased, and sitters interviewed and hired. Friends in his community responded to his need as he had responded to theirs for so many years. Some cooked. Some sat and talked. Others attended to problems around the house. Many volunteered to drive him to dialysis each Monday, Wednesday, and Friday. He could not have returned home without their assistance.

Though home, he talked even less. Conversation required energy, and he had little. Granddad had finally accepted that he would always require dialysis. From medication changes to blood tests to home health visits, all his care focused on managing his illness. His thoughts, however, seemed to be moving in a different direction, ahead of his family and physicians. When he was awake, which was never for long, he moaned quietly as he tried to shift his weight from side to side on the couch. But he was thinking, and he periodically shared his thoughts, usually in the form of questions. On a few occasions, he asked me about his options. He wanted to know if there were any other forms of treatment. Could he find relief from this "misery"? Did the dialysis have to be so painful? Did it have to be continued? What would happen if he stopped?

The conversations were difficult, and I did the best I could to answer his questions. He did not have the strength to talk for very long on any given occasion. My work and the distance between our homes limited the time we could spend together. His family, friends, nurses, and physicians all remained focused on his various illnesses as the list constantly increased. His attention, though, was focused on home—on staying home and on going "home." My grandfather was a man of faith. He did not fear death; he was prepared to die. In the private world of his thoughts and prayers, he seemed to have crossed a threshold. While all those around him labored to fix his broken story, he quietly began to draft its final chapter.

On October 22, 1996, the third day, the die was cast. My grandmother passed away in her sleep. When I heard, I was stunned. "Granny, not Granddad?" I asked my mother over the phone. No one expected her to go first, although she had some health concerns, as does almost everyone at age eighty-two. "How is Granddad?" I knew the answer but did not know what else to ask. His companion and best friend for the past sixty-one years was gone. We buried her two days later. He sat, in his wheelchair, among the hundreds of flower arrangements that encircled her grave, sad and deep in thought. Then he returned to his house—a house that was no longer a home without my grandmother. His decision was almost made, but he had three questions.

The day after my grandmother's funeral, we had our most detailed and significant conversation. He was scheduled to go for dialysis. "What will happen if I don't go back?" he asked.

"I don't know" was the only answer I could provide. I had never encountered this circumstance before. I knew he could delay his treatment a day, maybe two. A few days later, I spoke with a nephrologist in my community. She seemed very uncomfortable with the conversation and described the difficult deaths of two patients who chose to stop dialysis during her fellowship. Beyond that she offered little.

Granddad's second question: "Will I suffer?"

I explained that this would be a difficult journey, but that I would do everything possible to limit his suffering. He would struggle to breathe as the waste and water normally removed through dialysis backed up in his body. However, the correct doses of the right medication would limit his pain. I did not know how it would be for me or for my family. With his permission, I talked with my mother who spoke with her brother. Together, we cautiously made our way down a road none of us had traveled before. I did not know how we would care for him. Who would prescribe his medication? Who would administer it? Hospice services were unavailable in his community. His home health nurse was excellent but would need a physician to direct the care she would provide. I was willing, but would I be able? And, should I?

My grandfather's third question was even more difficult to address. "What about the 'suicide clause'?" I welcomed, with caution and awe, the privilege of discussing his concerns with him. I was not a philosopher, theologian, or ethicist. I was his grandson and a physician, and I was increasingly being asked to be *his* physician. This journey was moving into strange, new waters. As we talked, I was careful to go only as far as he went. I did not present new options. I sought to accompany him on his journey and assured him that I would remain at his side. We shared a faith tradition; one that he thought had a "suicide clause." Was this suicide? Was it prohibited? I did not think so. "Talk with others," I encouraged him. Not given to rash or hasty decisions, Granddad approached this decision in his usual careful and thoughtful manner.

We continued our conversation over the subsequent two weeks, and worked our way through the possible answers to each of his questions. We referenced the Christian Scriptures, talked about his relationship with God, and spoke of the confidence with which he felt he could approach the end of his life. We discussed other situations in which patients make decisions to withdraw life-sustaining medical care such as mechanical ventilation and tube feedings. He concluded that for him discontinuing renal dialysis was similar to discontinuing mechanical ventilation in the face of an irreversible, terminal illness. His kidneys had failed and would not recover. His life was without joy and now devoid of the experiences that had given it rich meaning for almost eight decades. Existence was limited to restless sleep on the bed or the sofa with painful, exhausting, and embarrassing trips to the bathroom.

As a family, we followed my grandfather across a threshold. He could not and would not write this chapter alone. My mother took an extended leave from her teaching position in Chicago and helped care for him. My uncle was more anxious; he wanted my grandfather to return to Nashville, be close by, and keep searching for the strength and desire to stay alive. However, both were willing to support whatever decision Granddad made.

After each conversation, I also spoke with a close friend and colleague who is a medical ethicist. I recreated each conversation for him, asking questions about the process and the issues. He questioned me about my thought, emotions, and intent. With his assistance, I tried to ensure that my ethical compass was frequently recalibrated. Without his assistance, I could not have continued.

My grandfather and I carefully worked through each of his questions. He seemed less concerned with gathering new information and more focused on confirming the decision he had made. "I'm not going back to dialysis any more," he said. He called his three surviving sisters and two nieces to his home to inform them of his decision and to say good-bye. Tuesday morning, the time for his next treatment, came and went. He stayed home on his couch with my mother at his side. He did not waver.

Signing the necessary papers, I assumed responsibility for my grandfather's care and became the attending physician of record. I discussed our plans with the home health nurse. A bedside suction was ordered. I would return for his final hours and administer the liquid morphine I would bring with me. He was still able to swallow, and he hated needles. We would not stick him again.

My grandfather's final three days were filled with special moments. He was surrounded by his family, who looked at pictures, told stories, and shared memories of my grandmother. Thursday morning he struggled to the table for a final meal of sausage, eggs, and tomatoes. He hesitated, remembering that he had not been allowed to eat tomatoes. When reassured, he winked, smiled, and enjoyed them.

When I arrived late Thursday night, he was awake. I sat beside him on the sofa, and we shared a bowl of banana pudding. He smiled reassuringly but did not say much. On Friday morning, we helped him from his bed to his couch and almost had to carry him. The deterioration overnight was remarkable. We took turns sitting on the floor beside him. I never moved farther than the next room. When needed, I suctioned the saliva from his mouth. When he awakened and groaned, I eased a spoonful of morphine into his mouth and wiped his lips. Initially I measured the volume and recorded the amount I gave him, but as the day wore on, this seemed unimportant.

Whenever he would awaken, someone was at his side to share the moment. His comments became less frequent and less coherent. He said, "So far, so good." and spoke of my grandmother, recalled his beloved mountains, and tried to sing a favorite hymn, "The Way of the Cross Leads Home." By the afternoon, he was much weaker and awake less often. "C'mon, let's go home," he said.

The morphine and the hypoxia-induced sleep kept him unaware of the fluid that was filling his lungs. "I'm ready. Let's go home," were his final words. He slept and did not arouse again. His son held one hand and his daughter the other. I moved across the room and sat in a chair, watching with quiet reverence. This location provided my parents, aunt, and uncle enough space to be at his side. Perhaps the move was symbolic as well. My grandfather was dying on the couch, but he was also my patient. I needed to maintain some space, to hold on to the *equinimitas* I had found. Until my task was completed, I wanted and needed to protect my objectivity.

The end came quietly. Some of those present had never witnessed a death before. Startled, they looked to me for an interpretation, a diagnosis, a verdict. My solemn nod unlocked the door to their grief. Together we—his family and friends, his church and community, and me as his grandson and physician—allowed my grandfather to go home and stay home. With grace and courage, he overcame the obstacles presented by the rural location where he lived. With hesitation and gratitude and with some sense of urgency and necessity, I overcame my uncertainty about the dual roles I was asked to play. I was honored and humbled by the privilege of helping my grandfather write the final chapter of his story. I believe he wrote it well.

Early Marriage: West Virginia

ANN FLOREEN NIEDRINGHAUS

I

The other nurses called them brambles:
prickly creepers climbing up the rock face.
Stopping the car I gathered
blackberries to make an offering
for you—crystal jelly, all seeds
strained out through a dish towel.
Patients warned me later, "You better
watch for copperheads on those cliffs."

You came home from hospital duty,
tired and distracted,
spread my ambrosia thickly and said,
I'd rather have Welch's.

II

Driving to home visits, I took as a road
a dry creek bed overhung
with branches and vines.
It ended at a sagging porch,
the family processed a pig,
newly slaughtered, on the kitchen table.
Drawing me in near the carcass,
folks spoke their maladies: *blind staggers,*
drizzlin' shits, a head gatherin'
that went away with *white lightnin'.*

And you walked home from your shift
in the emergency room
with your own stories: a man impaled

through the chest with a telephone pole,
a woman with a neck goiter the size
of a cantaloupe; a child
whose *smilin' mighty Jesus*
was spinal meningitis.
We talked in the dark before you fell asleep
feeling like Lewis and Clark.

III
Perched on the steepest hill in town,
our house was two stories high on the street,
four stories high in the back.
The gleaming Monongahela River
filled the winding valley bottom far below.

Years later my mother told us,
There was a hole in the bathroom wall.
I worried about rats.
We were surprised.
We couldn't remember a hole.

Teen Pregnancy: "We Were Hoping"

PATRICIA J. HARMAN

At 4:00 P.M. Dee Telemann is fifteen minutes late for her 3:45 appointment. It gives me a chance to return a few phone calls. It's a familiar last name, Telemann. She's probably the daughter of my patient, Sara, who lives on a farm out on Snake Run.

At 4:45, an hour overdue, the patient arrives with a boyfriend and a young child in tow. I stand from my desk, stretch and look out the window, out at the white clouds climbing like stair steps against the blue sky.

Spring, summer, and fall, Tom, my husband and practice partner, and I try to bicycle after work. I'm hoping this will be a quick visit so we can get out on the trail. Next to Dee's name, on the computer printout, it says only, "New GYN with personal concerns." *Personal concerns* is never a quick visit.

Striding down the hall, a little pissed, I reach the exam room door and tap twice. It's a utilitarian knock. I intend to get right down to business and set the girl straight on the importance of coming to appointments on time. Dee sits on the edge of the exam table, a petite blond with the smooth tan skin and high cheekbones of a lot of Appalachian women. She's dressed in jeans and a low-cut white blouse.

Her young man slouches in the gray guest chair in a T-shirt with some kind of motorcycle logo on it. He wears tight, worn jeans, a creased baseball cap, and run-down cowboy boots. It's an outfit I don't see much around Torrington where most of the young men wear hip-hop clothing, or what passes for it in the hills of West Virginia, baggy pants low on their hips, an oversized T-shirt and Kango hat. I know that look well. It's a style my sons perfected when they were in high school. In the man's lap sits a young boy with big ears, buzzed white-blond hair and a grin on his face.

"Hi, Dee, I'm Patsy Harman, nurse-midwife and GYN practitioner." I reach out my hand and note the girl's firm grip.

"I'm Tommy," the little boy says. "I'm her brother. I'm six." I shake his hand too. I'm surprised and a little uncomfortable that the youngster has been brought into the small exam room. Having a child present will make a GYN checkup more difficult.

"This is my boyfriend, Jerry," Dee says proudly. "My fiancé." Jerry nods and meets my eyes. He's a small guy, but muscular, about five feet nine with light brown hair curling over his shoulders. I glance at the birth date on the patient's chart. She's sixteen. He could be eighteen.

Because she was late, I'd been prepared to start off the encounter with a lecture about the importance of coming to appointments on time, but curiously I skip it. "So Dee, what brings you here today? Are you having difficulties?"

"Oh, no real problems. . . . We're just pregnant. We did *three* home tests." Her face glows and she looks at Jerry for confirmation. He grins but then quickly pulls a shade over his joy.

"Yeah," says the little boy, "They're going to have a *baby*. Dee Dee and Jerry sitting in a tree. K-I-S-S-I-N-G." He sings this last part.

Jerry puts his hand gently over the kid's mouth and says with a twang, "Hush, now." That's all he says and the boy shuts up. The young man shifts him onto his other knee and wraps his arms around him.

"So, is this a good thing that you're pregnant? A happy thing?" From the look that has just passed between the two lovers, it's obvious.

"Oh, yeah, we were hoping it would happen. The only problem is, we don't have any money or a medical card. I was hoping you would take care of me until I can get one. I wish you could deliver our baby too, but the receptionist said you don't anymore."

I hesitate before I explain, unsure if teenagers will understand, then apologetically, begin. "The malpractice insurance for doing obstetrics just got too high. Now we only do prenatal care. We liked delivering babies. My husband, Dr. Tom, and I were a team, but then one January the premiums for Obstetrics went from $70,000 to $130,000. We just couldn't do it. You can buy a pretty good house in Jefferson County for that amount, a house every year, that's what it amounts to."

Jerry gives a low whistle. They get the picture.

I narrow my eyes thinking about reimbursement. "Do your parents have health insurance?"

"I don't know, but if they do, it wouldn't cover me. I quit school."

I want to ask why she dropped out. She seems smart enough, but I stick to the subject. There will be time for that later. "Have you applied for medical assistance?"

"Not yet. We need my mom's signature or a health care provider to verify that I'm pregnant. I was thinking that could be *you*. . . . We need a due date too, on the form." She stops. They all stare at me.

"Does your Mom *know* you're pregnant?"

"Not yet. We wanted to wait until Jerry gets his first paycheck from Taco Bell so she'll see we can be responsible. She doesn't even know I came to see you."

Sara Telemann, married, thirty-four, a rural postal carrier, has eight children. I delivered the last one, and Tom did her tubal. Will she be happy when she finds out the news? Does she expect her daughter to get pregnant early and often? Or will she be angry seeing Dee repeat the old pattern?

I glance over the new OB intake form. The girl is low risk. Like most teenagers, she hasn't been around long enough to have many medical problems. After a quick physical and a review of the OB packet, I take them all down the hall to the ultrasound room. Standing in the dark, I point out the tiny fetus on the monitor. It's just eight weeks, but it has arms and legs and there's a flicker of a fetal heartbeat. "I'm your uncle," the little boy announces, touching the screen with his finger. Dee has tears in her eyes, and Jerry reaches over to touch her bare foot. I give them a picture of the baby and a copy for the little boy too.

"Now don't you go telling Mom?" Dee Dee threatens.

"He won't or he'll be sorry," Jerry says, rubbing the kid's fuzzy head.

In the end, I sign the papers for the medical card and tell the young woman to call the welfare office first thing in the morning. "And I want you to tell your mom about the pregnancy before your next appointment. Legally I can take care of you as an 'emancipated minor,' but I would prefer it to be out in the open." I don't say, "Because if your mom comes to see me, you may meet one day in the waiting room."

Dee and Jerry will be good parents. Maybe they'll be parents of eight like Sara. Their children will be responsible, well behaved, and loving like Sara's and get pregnant at sixteen or seventeen and have more babies. They'll work at Taco Bell or Wal-Mart or Select Tech, the telemarketing place downtown. Maybe one or two will stay on the farm or go to community college for nursing or computers.

Standing at the check out desk, I watch the young couple leave with arms wrapped around each other. They have everything against them—youth, poverty, and lack of education—but they love each other and seem so solid. I think of a mountain covered with trees.

Indian Dinner in Johnson City

ABRAHAM VERGHESE

Rajani and I made our way to the party that was being held in the gym of a local school, the Ashley Academy. We were quite late.

The Ashley parking lot was full: a few Honda Civics, an abundance of Honda Accords, a few minivans, a few Acuras (a natural progression from an Accord), and one Mercedes-Benz were in the lot.

The Indian community in Johnson City was growing logarithmically. The new complement of interns and residents always included three or more Indians, most of them married, some with children. They were the friends, relatives or classmates of those who had gone through the ETSU residency program, people who now put them up, lent them the rule book to study for the Tennessee driving license exam, shepherded them to the Highway Patrol office to take the test, cosigned their loan for the Honda Civic, helped them find an apartment, instructed them on whether the vegetables were fresher at Kroger's or Winn Dixie's, and introduced them to the old-timers of Johnson City, like Rajani and myself.

Once the newcomers were settled, they expressed their gratitude by inviting their mentors and their mentors' friends over for a grand dinner. The mentors, once newcomers themselves, now had moved one step closer to the inner stratum of the social circle. At its center were a patriarchal group of families who had been there before the medical school and before liquor-by-the-drink had come to town. They had been there when North Roan Street was the edge of town; they were there before the mall, the banks, the car dealers, and the little strip malls with their necklace of colorful awnings had arrived on North Roan. Like a water beetle, the new development on North Roan had sucked the life out of downtown, leaving only a carcass. The old-timers told us how beautiful and quaint downtown had been: the Majestic Theater, the Fountain Plaza. . . . Now it was an empty shell of a business area with a few boutiques displaying slope-shouldered mannequins in faded and dusty fashions from the fifties.

Texas Instruments and Eastman-Kodak also brought in a regular crop of engineers of Indian origin. These "techie" types, when I saw them at a party, always struck me as unused to the bright glare of the outside world, staring out at it ferretlike. After four years of cracking books in the library of some state university (those at Amherst and Buffalo were especially popular) and skewing the grade curve in a manner to make things impossible for their American student peers (who still held dear the three Fs of college life—fraternities, football, and frolicking with the opposite sex), they appeared quite lost.

Meanwhile, more foreign doctors were setting up practice in the smallest towns of rural Tennessee, southwest Virginia, and Kentucky after completing their training in an urban residency. They made expeditions to our provincial metropolises of Johnson City, Kingsport and Bristol—the Tri-Cities—to do their shopping, to look up families that were friends of friends of friends, and to gradually become regulars at any of the major functions, such as Dipavali or Indian Independence Day, that justified an excursion of such length.

New York City and Chicago had long gotten used to the sight of Indians manning newspaper kiosks, driving cabs, running gas stations, working as staff nurses or doctors in the metropolitan hospitals, and even trying their hand at the pretzel and hot dog concessions. And now, the glittery variety shops that were once the province of the Lebanese, the Yemenis, and the Jews had competition from Indians. Indians had learned the art of cramming the window displays with autofocus cameras, palm-sized cameras, video cameras, 8-mm cine cameras, hand-held televisions, car televisions, stereos, VCRs, CDs, radios, two-in-one boom boxes, three-in-ones, four-in-ones, five-in-ones, computers, calculators, pens, time managers, wristwatches, pen-size dictaphones, strobe lights, binoculars, telephoto lenses, tripods, telescopes, and lava lamps. This phantasmagoria was peppered with SALE! SALE! banners and little fold-up cards sat below each item with the "price" prominently displayed in fluorescent green, yellow and red, below the crossed-out "retail" price. It was as difficult for a grown man to walk past such a store as it was to whisk a child through Toys "R" Us without stopping. And once you were caught by this display, transfixed by the stare of the hundred lenses, captured by the four video cameras that now projected your image onto every TV screen in that window—shopper transformed into variety store star—you became like a deer trapped in a hunter's flashlight.

The dark-skinned man at the door, with hair curling out of his shirt collar and peeping out at his wrists, watched you, smiled easily, nodded to his assistant who mysteriously appeared with the *one* item that had tugged at you. As he ushered you into the interior of the shop, where incense burned at the foot of idols of Lakshmi and Ganesh, he reminded you how indispensable a pair of binoculars with power-zoom was to a citizen of the world.

These visible Indians in the big city were but a fraction of the total number of Indians that lived there, worked quietly as accountants, engineers, Port Authority workers, students, computer programmers, immigration officials . . .

In a town our size, without the very visible trades of taxi drivers or newspaper *wallahs* to use as a yardstick, it was tricky to establish exactly how many Indians there were. My friend Brij, a traveling Hong-Kong-suit salesman (the kind who will set up his tie and shirt displays on the ground floor of an Embassy Suites for a day, run advertisements in the local paper, and then take orders for custom-tailored suits which are stitched in Hong-Kong, by Indians, and mailed back in a week), describes his foolproof method of gauging the local Indian population and finding an Indian restaurant in a strange city:

"You look in white pages under B for 'Bombay Palace' or T for 'Taj Mahal' or I for 'India House.' These are equivalent of Asia Palace, Bamboo House, China Garden, or House of Hunan in the Chinese restaurant business. If there are no listings under those names, take my word there are probably no Indian restaurants in town. Failing this, you simply look up number of Patels in white pages and multiply by 60; that will tell you size of Indian community, *not* counting wives, children and in-laws. Take my word: less than ten Patels means no Indian restaurant. If more than ten, you call, say you are from India, ask them where to go to eat."

"But, Brij," I asked. "Why don't you just look under 'Restaurants' in the Yellow Pages?"

"*Aare*, that's no fun, *yar!*"

Even if it was not readily measured, Indianization, the entrepreneurial spirit of the variety store, was trickling out to the hinterland. The sari shops, the video stores, and the spice shops in New York, Atlanta, and Chicago were now into mail-order. Indian culture was following on the heels of the Coca-Cola truck, going wherever it went, probing deep into rural America. A Gujarati couple from Charlotte sent flyers out in the mail to announce the days they would be in Johnson City. The flyer listed their complete itinerary which, much like the itinerary of a country singer, began in Charlotte and took them up to Boone, North Carolina; Johnson City, Tennessee; Bristol, Virginia, and Bristol, Tennessee; Wise, Virginia, and then back home.

In Johnson City, they parked their van at the former Mid-Town Inn, with the blessing of the new Indian owners. Along the insides of their Ford van they had rigged up crude shelves. The floor of the van was loaded with giant sacks of basmathi rice, raw rice, rice flour, lentils, and a balancing pan to weigh out the rice. In the recesses of the van were bottles of Ambedkar mango and lime pickles and *papads*. They carried the complete product line of the Surati Sweet Mart, a company with offices in Toronto, Ontario, and River Rouge, Michigan. Surati Sweet Mart produced a line of packaged and canned goods that included *badam puree, barfi, badampak, bundi ladu, farsi puree, gulab jambu, ghari, jalebi, khaman, khajili, kachori, mesub, mohan thal, penda, surti bhusu, chevdo, sev* and *gathiya.*

The wife, a formidable lady with a giant diamond in her nose, thick gold bangles on her wrists and a no-nonsense air about her, sat on the lip of the cargo space, further jeopardizing the van's suspension. Her hand rested possessively on the weighing machine. If you requested an item other than rice or flour or lentils, she yelled the order to her husband, a thin individual who never emerged from the recess of the van, but stayed crouched in the back. You only saw his gangly arms handing out items to his wife. Her size precluded her from fulfilling this task.

The parking lot was full of doctors and engineers. I spoke no Hindi and the Gujarati couple spoke no Tamil or Malayalam, so when it came my turn, we carried out our transactions there in the former Mid-Town Inn parking lot in English:

"Three packets of *papads*—"

"Plain or chili?"

"Chili. And two kilos of basmathi rice—"

"I give you discount on five kilos."

A new fad had swept the Johnson City Indian community. Instead of inviting people to each other's houses for dinner, families were renting out the gym of the Ashley Academy, a private school, to host dinner for sixty to a hundred people. In one fell swoop, a family could reciprocate for every dinner they had been invited to over the previous year. In doing so they also racked up the certainty of invitations for the rest of the year, a year that could be spent at leisure until they were in the debit column again.

As more families followed this trend, the dinners took on a surreal quality: the same gym, the same crowd, almost the same food—only the host changed.

Rajani and I stepped inside the gym. The women had, as usual, gravitated to one side, the men to the other, and children were playing noisily in the middle. There was a constant din in the room from all the voices.

I moved around the room greeting people I had seen just two weeks ago in the same gym.

This party, like every other such party, was "dry"—no alcohol was served. This was in itself curious, as I had never known any of these hosts to decline my scotch or gin or rum at our house. Of course, a "dry" dinner could be thought of as being more traditional, like in the old country. But here in this prep school gym, children running around with ninja figures and robot transformers in their hands, the most fluent east Tennessee patois rolling off the tongues of toddlers and teens alike, it was difficult to invoke the old country, difficult to ascribe the "dry" dinners to anything but an unbecoming miserliness.

I looked around the room and saw Rajani with a group of fifteen women, all of them, including Rajani, wearing colorful saris, or *salwar-kamiz*, all of them sitting on the gym benches and chatting. The different states of India that were revealed in subtle aspects of dress and jewelry included Maharashtra, Andhra Pradesh, Uttar Pradesh, Punjab, Tamil Nadu, Kerala, and Orissa; there were an equal number of unique dialects. English was the only language common to all. Rajani was laughing and enjoying herself in a way that I hadn't seen for a long time. Another group of women with a few men were helping the hostess bring the food (prepared at home over the past few days) in the giant cooking pots to the row of tables strung end to end to make a buffet table.

The teenage girls buzzed and whispered together, staying in their one geographic spot all night. The teenage boys stood sullen together, on the men's side of the room. They looked displeased at being made to come to these functions.

Among the men, the pecking order at these functions was clear: doctors ruled over engineers, who lorded it over everyone else. The motel owner's status depended on how successful he was as an entrepreneur. But then financial success was really at the root of the hierarchy among the doctors: surgeons—particularly thoracic surgeons—were treated as the maharajahs, everyone rising when this persona entered the room. Plastic surgery and urology were a notch below thoracic surgery. (And even if the urologist made more money, there was something just a little unclean about the idea of urology—it had tinges of untouchability, what with working with urine and all that.) Then followed the cardiologists and the gastroenterologists and the other *procedural* medical specialists. Needless to say, on this ranking, being an infectious diseases specialist was equivalent to being a bathroom sweeper.

To have made the choice of the specialty of infectious diseases was, in this circle, considered akin to buying at full price a motel that any Patel could have told you was going belly-up and that you could have bought for a *bhajan* at foreclosure.

Tonight, as always, I was the recipient of much advice. Most of it was on how to make money, since I clearly wasn't making any. In the competition to build a larger and fancier house, I was not even in the race: I was *renting* from the VA—a heinous crime from the perspective of an Indian community that saw land acquisition as a primal necessity. ("But what about my oak trees?" I wanted to say. "What about the bed of red salvia I have in front? What about the yellow and red roses? What about my tomatoes?" I knew the answer: it would be "What about equity?")

I acted as if money meant less to me than it did to them, a childish reflex. This was, of course, not true: I valued money and would not have minded a ton of it. But I didn't feel I had to do something different in medicine *just* for that reason. I was every bit as well trained, just as talented I like to think, as the doctors who made twenty times what I made. The monetary disparity was not due to their skill or their intrinsic worth (even though at times I think they succumbed to this delusion); it was due to a payment system that placed greater value on procedural specialties than on those without them.

"Ah, but in *Sweden*," I would say when I grew tired of being needled about my specialty, "thoracic surgeons and infectious diseases specialists get the same salary. And you know what, if the *Democrats* win the next election . . ."

This was guaranteed to produce a loud outcry that I delighted in. There were no stauncher Republicans than the Indian doctors of east Tennessee.

I tired of this after a while, tired of the talk of stock options and mutual funds and the benefits of incorporating. I drifted over to the teenage boys. To them I was a hero of sorts. Not only did I *not* drive a Honda Accord, not only had I *never* owned a new car, I even owned a motorcycle and rode it when the weather permitted. I took them for rides, not necessarily with their parents' knowledge. And on top of that, I took care of AIDS patients! Whatever it was their daddies did, there was no personal danger. In truth, there was no personal danger in what I did, but that evening I did not fight the St. George-the-dragon-slayer metaphor.

With a little encouragement, I found myself waxing eloquent about AIDS care, telling them how it enriched my life, changed its direction. Some of the teenage girls shuffled over. I marshaled a passionate argument against Reagan, deliberately planting a seed of dissension in their family. I told them a risqué joke: how the urologist who removed Reagan's prostate was asked later by Reagan if all was well, would the plumbing now work well? "Everything is perfect. Your bladder is fine. Your penis is one-hundred percent. You can go out and fuck the country for another four years!" The loud laughter drew looks from the parents.

As I talked to the teenagers, I was conscious that my words created a reality far superior to the actual reality of what I did. But the teens were chiming in now: they had such pure ideas of justice, of right and wrong, of what they would do if they were in control. I loved it! If their parents were the ultimate pragmatists, these kids were beautiful idealists.

When the summons for dinner came, and the line started to form to walk past the table and pick up the pooris, the channa, the rice, the vegetable curry, the pickle, the yogurt and the sweet, our little group broke up. Children went first. I picked up my paper plate and stood with the ranks of the men. By long-standing Ashley Academy Indian dinner tradition—a token concession to years of oppression—the men would serve themselves *after* the women.

An hour or two later, I was ready to leave. I thanked our host. Looking for Rajani, I approached the side of the room where the women were sitting. A father stopped me, his expression half-serious, half-joking. He said he was mortified to hear his daughter say to him a few minutes ago that when she finished medical school (and these kids were all going into medical school, even the ten-year-olds), she thought she would become an AIDS specialist.

I shook his hand and offered him my warmest congratulations and turned away. Ahead of me I could see Rajani, still laughing, at the center of a circle of women. She seemed perfectly at home. I didn't want to take her away.

This selection is chapter 11 in Abraham Varghese's *My Own Country: A Doctor's Story of a Town and Its People in the Age of AIDS* (New York: Simon & Schuster, 1994).

White Coat at Midnight

RICHARD M. BERLIN

This morning my best friend
will come with his chain saw
and ax, and we'll cut down
the ash where a barred owl
perched last night and hooted
his four note song. We'll split it
and stack it into cords, and I'll be
thinking about midnight
in January when the air is twenty
below zero and the northern
lights shimmer purple and blue.
My Defiant woodstove will be
burning today's work at 700,
and I'll be warm enough to open
a window wide and listen
again for owls and the calls
of coyotes yipping at the moon,
my monogrammed white coat
draped on a peg, washed
whiter by the moonlight,
hanging around for the next
moment of healing, like winter
waiting for the earth's heart to thaw.

Where We Are

Where We Are—Synopsis

TOM BIBEY

We are rural. The landscape may be in evolution, but some things never change. Spring planting will come around every year, and some of our patients will sit on the front porch and smoke cigarettes because that is what they do. Yeah, our patients eat too much at times and don't exercise enough, and maybe they aren't all that sophisticated, but don't diss 'em. They are our patients. We are them, and they are us. We don't talk bad about our own.

For us, a fragrance reminiscent of childhood will forever be spring rain and dandelions rather than Vicks VapoRub and BENGAY. There is nothing wrong with the folks who grew up in the city, they just missed those things. It can only enter the subconscious if you were raised with it.

Dr. Cohen might just as well have written about my office as his own. Has he been here? Mine is just down from the liquor store too. The floors slope and the roof leaks much like his. We don't have enough money for a new one either. Lord, Dr. Cohen, we're with you. Stylish? Trendy? Well, let's just say *Southern Living* ain't been by to profile our crib yet, and I don't look for 'em anytime soon.

As rural docs, we'll always live with our people. I'll bet Dr. Cohen is just like me. My guess is when he goes to the grocery store his patients look in his cart to see if he buys the same food he tells them to eat.

And yet before you misunderstand, let me reassure. We are modern. We use the same medicines as our city counterparts, and we are only a helicopter flight away from the latest technology, not that it solves all of our problems. We take the same competency tests as our colleagues, and I'll bet we do just as well or better. (Maybe my old professors did a little better, but they got to write the questions.) We have access to the same information too. My computer is just as fast as the ones over in Raleigh.

We've been around long enough to see the trends come and go. I've seen Aldactone fall in and out of favor three times now as the latest "hip" drug. When I see some young fellow tout the latest study on the merits of the drug as some new thing, I ache from his lack of wisdom.

The folks who have coexisted with the land for centuries have more answers than we give them credit for. Modern thought on the best approach to the diagnosis of prostate cancer is a good example. The "correct" answers to the test questions "change." "What is the best screening test for prostate cancer?" The answer used to be "the rectal exam," then changed to "the PSA." Now it is "informed consent with the patient at risk for prostate cancer as to the risk vs. benefit of screening studies." (I thought this was what is had been all along.) On the next board exam I'd predict the correct response will be "do nothing," at least if the bean counters have their way.

Dr. Connolly's Navajo patients have known the correct answer to the questions for years— they never changed; folks just didn't listen like they should have. And I'll bet the Amish folks Dr. Kroening delivers are no worse off as a society for a low C-section rate modern docs have tried to find their way back to.

As rural docs, we at least deserve this much credit. We not only listen to our patients' points of view, we respect those views. As Dr. Loxterkamp says, we are connected; we live with our people. We are codependent with them and listen that we all might survive.

Years ago, I lost an elderly patient. The man was eighty-five, and had end-stage aortic stenosis. As my consultants began to sign off the case, I realized the end was near. All docs know end-stage aortic valve disease can be ugly—he all but drowned. In the end, tears and morphine were all I had to offer, about the same treatment they would have used in Civil War days. After he was gone, I sat at the bedside and pondered it. An old doc came by and put his arm around my shoulder.

"You did everything you could, Bibey."

"Hell, Dr. Robbins, I didn't do anything. I just had to sit there and watch the man die. They wasn't nothing I could do," I said.

"Oh yes, there was, Bibey. You were there. Sometimes all we can do is show up, and you did that. It was all you could do."

I never forgot his words. When everyone else drops away and I'm the last doc left, I know the end is near, and I show up. At times it might be all we have left to do, but that's what rural docs do.

Our technology will evolve and it will help us, but it will never replace the heart and soul of rural doctors. I depend on my patients to fix my car or cut my hair. They depend on me to doctor them just like their parents and grandparents did before them. You don't have to ask the family history if you were there.

If I live long enough, though, there will come a day when my people will go to a diagnostic center at the mall where some computer will prick their finger, render an opinion, and spit out a few pills for them to take.

When that happens they are still going to call me, or someone like Dr. Cohen, and ask, "Doc, this here computer at the mall gave me these blue pills. You reckon they'll do me any good?"

And I'm gonna say, "Well, Joe, I don't know. What kinda trouble you having? Maybe you better come over to the office and let me take a look. It's closed right now. You just meet me at the back door and . . ."

Spring Planting

RICHARD M. BERLIN

For Julianna A. Luntz Van Raan, 1950–1998

A morning call wakes me:
something hard and fibrous in her leg
growing fast and uncontrolled
that can't be weeded out.
Through my bedroom window
I study winter rye in April
swinging on strong stems.
I wish I could plant Julie's leg
in a warm tangle of earth,
turn her face toward the sun,
and let her nurse on spring rain
like the dandelions waiting
to fill the meadow with stars.

Welcome to Elma

MITCHELL L. COHEN

Hey, you must be our medical student for the day. Short white coat gave it away. Did you find the office OK? Good, directions aren't too difficult. There's only one light in town and I always tell people if you just look for the funeral home and the liquor store we're just past that. People often drive right past the building though. Most think it is just a one-floor rambler style house. They really have no idea of the history of what's happened here.

So you're here for one day during your family medicine rotation. Don't worry too much about learning about how to manage congestive heart failure or pneumonia. Maybe you'll pick up a tip or two. But, you're job for the day is to see what the life of a small-town family doctor is like. This may be your only opportunity to see what rural medicine is all about. It's a chance to see how things are done when there isn't an MRI down the hall or dozens of subspecialists over in the next office. It's your chance to see what it's like to care for large families and to have them think of you as "the doctor." I'll give you a tour of the office and then we'll have you see some patients.

Come down the hall this way; let me show you this picture. This is a drawing of this office back when it was a hospital. It was built in 1898 by Dr. Blair. There were two beds for men, two for women, and a surgery/storage area. The nurses lived in a house attached at this end. Did I mention there was no running water or electricity when he opened his hospital? He put that in ten or twenty years later.

You saw the waiting room when you came in. We're always debating the wood paneling on the walls. It's not the most stylish or trendy thing for waiting rooms, and some people think it's outright ugly, but I have to admit I'm kind of attached to it. This community was built on logging, and it only seems right to have wood paneling in the waiting room.

Up here we have the nurses' area to weigh people, check blood pressures, get immunizations ready, and what not. We had to buy a new scale recently. The old one, which dated back to when the building was a hospital, only went up to three hundred pounds. This new one accommodates more of our population now. It's not your imagination: the floor is really slanted at the corner there.

The roof leaks around the gutters and the ground is starting to sink from being saturated. It's almost like the rain water intentionally avoids the gutter. We really need to fix up this building or get a new one, but the money for that has to come from somewhere.

Moving on down the hall are my partners' offices. Have you met them yet? They are both women who choose to work part time to help balance being doctors and moms. I'm sure Dr. Blair never thought that there would be two women, not to mention two mothers, working here as physicians. Sometimes things do change for the better.

You also might notice that these offices are the size of a walk-in closet, and yet my partners have their desks right next to their nurses. We're definitely a close-knit family here, and sometimes we probably take it to an extreme. We're not terribly formal, and we have very few written rules. Despite this, and maybe because of this, we have the best staff anyone could want. This is their practice as much as it is ours. All of the staff has been here longer than I have, and most staff members are patients here too, as are their families. My nurse, who's fifty (shhhh! don't tell her I told you), has her childhood immunization records in her chart here. You just don't find this kind of environment in your urban or suburban large multispecialty clinic where the staff is just there punching their time cards.

The exam rooms here are as obscenely tiny as the offices. To tell you the truth, I'm not sure how these rooms ever functioned as hospital rooms. I measured them once and they come to be about six by fifteen feet. Wait until you try to do a Pap smear in one of them—quite the challenge. We have three general exam rooms and one that we've made a little more kid friendly.

See that sign above the door down there marked "Emergency"? Let's go in there. Back when this was a hospital, this was the emergency room, and we still refer to it as the ER. The back door still has the sign saying "Emergency Entrance Only" on it. It's been a long time since an ambulance rolled up here, but the ER makes for a nice procedure room. We do your basic "lumps and bumps" here—skin biopsies, remove cysts, sew up lacerations from time to time. It's also a nice room to do casting and splinting. All of those metal bedpans and glass urinals on the shelf over there are from the original hospital.

Moving on down to the other end of the hallway in between the ER and the "emergency entrance" is a kitchen. Patient meals were made here once upon a time. You see, however, that the glass cabinets that once held plates, bowls, and glasses are now filled with rows of bins of drug samples. I always wonder what the old-time doctors would have thought of this. Would they have been amazed at so many options for medications, or would they have been disgusted by the big business medicine has turned into? I tend to think "yes" to both.

OK, let's move back to the end of the building. Here's the minilibrary we've built and a computer that you're free to use. We're still fairly technologically challenged out here. Our IT department consists of whatever we can figure out or con friends and family into helping us with.

Information technology is certainly one of the biggest challenges of being in a small, rural practice. There's so much potential yet so many barriers. Purchasing, implementing, and maintaining an electronic health record is an expensive proposition. Telemedicine could help bring specialists in for virtual office visits, but again, who can afford to set that up? There's admittedly some element of technophobia in here. Much of our staff, as wonderful as they are, still is not comfortable with some basic computer functions. There's a certain conservatism that comes with small-town life, and while this is often a good thing, technophobia is probably not good.

The last room in the building is our X-ray area. Some say that there's a ghost, a blue woman who people think worked here as a nurse. I don't know, never had a sighting myself, but just ask some of the nurses. As you can see from all of the boxes filled with patient charts on the table, we haven't done an X-ray in this building in over ten years. For such a small practice it just hasn't been cost effective. For imaging we send people ten miles up the road for an X-ray at our local critical access hospital. They just got a CT scanner there as well, which we're all very excited about. However, if patients need ultrasound or MRI, they have to travel thirty miles to the referral hospital for our five-county region. The roof is leaking back here too. It just goes around the gutters; wish the ghost would repair it.

Here's a list of the patients we'll be seeing today. I like to describe our patients as a mix of "Rockwell" versus "Red Neck." On the one hand, many are somewhat humble, hard working, and friendly who look like they posed for Norman Rockwell. On the other hand, there are your stereotypical uneducated, overweight people who sit on the porch of their trailers smoking cigarettes.

My partners and I are the only doctors for a fifty-mile stretch of highway to provide maternity care. It's a service for patients and it brings kids into our practices. About 20 to 25 percent of the patients are kids. As far as the adult patients go, it's as challenging and complicated a group as you'd find in any internal medicine practice. We do a lot of mental health care as well. There's one part-time psychiatric nurse practitioner for the entire county, so we save our toughest psychiatric cases for her, while we handle the rest.

First on the schedule is a forty-year-old log truck driver coming in to get his physical for his license. I never knew how many log truck drivers were in this county until I started working here. Here's a thirty-two-year-old female with chest pain that's probably caused by either her asthma, anxiety, or both. She smokes way too much tobacco and marijuana. Then there's a depressed patient with fairly newly diagnosed diabetes, high blood pressure, and elevated cholesterol. It's so frustrating. He just doesn't seem to care, but I know a lot of this is the depression. The next guy you've got to meet. He is eighty-nine and coming in to talk about his gout. He's a retired veterinarian and tells some pretty amazing stories. Just ask him about serving in Italy in World War II. A tough case is next: an ADHD kid in foster care. We'll do a skin biopsy on the next guy. His dad is one of my patients in the nursing home. Really sad; rapidly advancing dementia. He's having a tough time watching his father go through so much.

Then it's lunchtime. Do you like Mexican food? Good. For lunch we'll walk over to this great Mexican place on the next block. The owners and most of the employees come here for their medical care too. I highly recommend the spinach enchilada.

In the afternoon we'll start with a pregnant patient of mine. I delivered her last baby. I also take care of her parents and grandparents. We have quite a few three- and four-generation families in the practice. My partner holds the record for a five-generation family, but then the great-great grandparent died and it went back to four generations. This guy here always comes in to get his ear wax cleaned out. Ahh, fascinating stuff there! Here's a guy in his mid-forties with low back pain and, and, oh by the way, he's seventy pounds overweight, smokes, and uses walking to his mailbox as his form of exercise. These visits are painful for both of us. Anyway, dispersed among all of those there are a few well-child visits, other pregnancy appointments, some of these might be Spanish speakers. How's your Spanish? I spent two years of my CME time leaning Spanish. I am passable, unless it gets complicated, then I use a phone translator—but as you'll learn, the visit fee hardly pays the cost. Then of course, more high blood pressure and diabetes, and the rest we'll figure out when we take a look on the other side of the door. Looks like about twenty-two patients total—pretty typical day.

Remember, you're here to learn about rural medicine. Get to know the patients. Let them tell you about their families and what they do for a living. You'll see that so much of what they tell you relates to their medical illnesses in ways that you haven't ever considered. This is one of the intangible benefits of family medicine, and it is best brought out in rural areas. It doesn't appear in any proficiency scores or quality measures, but the continuity of care we provide for generations of families allows us to tailor modern medicine to fit their needs. This is the art of medicine.

Any questions? Let's get you started here then. Here, go see this log truck driver. Welcome to town!

DINE: Navajo, *People*

MAUREEN CONNOLLY

Tsaile is cool at five thousand feet,
little snow, lots of space.

Weekdays I rise in the dark, watch the sun
bleed across the Lukachukai Mountains
out my kitchen window.
I see patients in the Indian Health Center:
pregnant women, diabetics, old women
in long skirts and velvet blouses, infants
brought in on cradleboards, injured men.

I learn how to speak some Navajo
how to listen to what is not said.
At the end of the day I walk outdoors
to where I sleep in the compound
near the dwellings of the other doctor
and the nurses. On the other side
of my little house, the sun bleeds
purple and orange over a pearled sky.

Once a week, I drive a winding road
into the dust and mud of Chinle
to a tiny emergency room bulging
with people. This winter babies
on the reservation are having trouble
breathing. There aren't enough beds.

Friday nights at the trading post,
I look at axes in a barrel, consider
popcorn versus pretzels, pick up

a free copy of the *Navajo Times*.
Weekends I hike the canyons.

In Window Rock I go to a rodeo
for the first time, sit on rough
planks in the stands, a white
woman alone among the Navajo.
Mothers put fry bread in toddler
mouths. Prepubescent girls eye
cowboys walking to the chutes
spurs glinting on their boots.
Boys enter on bucking calves
then grown men clinging to huge steers.

Clowns open gates, tempt belligerent
animals away from fallen riders,
know that elusive thing, when
to step out of the line of danger.
I leave early, fearful of livestock
or a drunken driver wandering
into my headlights on the dark
journey through the mountains.

I attend mass in a hogan-shaped
church, its curved inside walls shared
by St. Francis and the corn goddess.
Statues of a medicine woman and man
stand alongside the Nativity crèche.
I discover the Irish and Navajo have
nearly the same word for "people."

The night before I am to go home
it snows for hours into the quiet.
By morning the mountain passes
near Tsaile are closed. I head my
rented sedan the opposite direction
from the airport in Albuquerque
in hopes of circling back.

In Navajo country a milk-blue sky
blurs into rich cream land,
rust-red canyons claimed
by the snow. A brindled horse,
breath foggy in the air, stands still,
ears erect, against the horizon.
The landscape, impossibly, expands.

Two jeeps appear, one before
me, one behind, angel me
a hundred miles, no other
vehicles in sight, past scattered
Navajo villages, above the timberline,
over a mountain. I slide
onto the interstate, the jeeps are gone.

Near Gallup I stop at a convenience
store, dizzied by its repleteness.
Albuquerque can only be entered
from the west, they say, the snow.
I am coming from the west. I aim
for Albuquerque, home, my lover.

Then the airport and a plane that will fly.
More people, things, speed, sound.
A prayer forms itself.
I continue to move in and out of danger.

Learning from an Amish Birth

EMILY KROENING

Finally the day was done; I'd been up thirty-six hours and could not bear the thought of doing one more thing . . . my cell phone chimed. Rita, the midwife said, "One of the Amish families is in labor at home. They usually go quickly. Meet me in the hospital parking lot; I'll be loading my blue van."

Twilight yielded to darkness, as Rita and I followed the four-lane asphalt road through town, merged to two-lane blacktop, then twisted through a network of gravel roads. The night was inky black; no moon, no stars, only the occasional spotlight at an "English" farm. The agreement between the Amish community and the clinic was that if an Amish woman would come into the clinic for an initial prenatal visit, then she would receive home visits from the midwives for the duration of her pregnancy and could deliver at home as long as there were no complications. Women who had several children often had an Amish lay midwife handle the delivery. "But we are the couple's quick transportation to the hospital if something goes wrong," Rita said. "Since Amish don't have phones, someone has to run to a neighbor's to call for help. Otherwise it's horse and buggy."

Rita turned her van into a farm and the headlights outlined a small frame house. A lantern's golden glow lit the front window. "Watch your step," Rita warned. I stepped cautiously over frozen piles of horse manure and jagged ruts in the driveway as we unloaded the van, stacking our tubs on the front porch. Herman, the husband, welcomed us at the door. He was tall and muscular, his woolly beard stretched past his collar. We wiped our feet on a small doormat and entered the kitchen. The house smelled like supper, something with tomatoes and onions. A wood stove, with a pile of logs nearby, radiated a toasty warmth. Rita introduced me to Ann, who labored in the rocking chair next to the stove. She wore a white linen gown, the typical undergarment, and a white bonnet, a kapp. Her mother was busy drawing water for tea from the pump that protruded from the corner of the cement kitchen floor. Edward, Herman and Ann's one-year-old son, hid among the folds of his grandmother's traditional blue dress.

Rita and I accompanied Ann into the adjoining bedroom. A double bed with a rough wooden headboard, an oak dresser with an oil lamp, and the baby crib were tucked into the small space. Herman had built the crib for Edward.

After checking her vitals, I helped Ann stretch out on the bed. Her uterus tightened with a contraction. Rita reassured Ann that her contractions were good. We listened for the familiar dlup, dlup, dlup . . . of the baby's heartbeat. A rate of 140, perfect. I gloved my hand and checked Ann's cervix. It was open to three centimeters and the length had thinned halfway. This would be a long night, but the novelty held my weariness at bay.

The bedroom was pleasantly warm. An alarm clock perched on the dresser cast a monumental shadow on the wall. Rita handed it to me and told me to set the alarm every fifteen minutes, the interval for checking the baby's heartbeat. The clock was the old-fashioned kind with a large clock face and metal ringer on the top. The key in the back grated as I wound it, setting the time: 8:30. Its soft ticking faded into background as we set up our theater: baby pack, instrument pack, sterile gloves, oxygen—just in case. We lay a plastic sheet over the mattress, letting it drape to the floor and covered it with towels.

We settled into routine. Grandmother entertained Edward and busied herself around the kitchen where Herman rested in a rocker near the stove with Rita nearby in a straight-back chair. In between contractions Ann and I talked about our lives. We were the same age—twenty-four. Ann took off her kapp and pulled pins from her coiled hair, releasing long blonde curls much like my own. Although they spoke German at home, Ann's English had only the hint of an accent. Born down the road, she attended school through eighth grade. Then she worked for a neighboring family as a helper, caring for children and assisting with household chores. "Are you married?" she asked me.

I shook my head. "Right now my focus is to get through medical school. Then maybe I'll have time to think about having a family."

The metallic bell of the alarm clock interrupted our conversation. Rita peered in while I listened for the baby's heartbeat. It continued to be strong. With an intense contraction, Ann moved onto her hands and knees. Laboring quietly and moaning occasionally, she did not ask for pain meds. After each contraction, I wiped her forehead with a washcloth, then massaged her boney shoulders, ropey biceps, and firm back. She was smaller than I, probably stronger as well, from physical labor. She talked of doing laundry in tubs by hand and tending the garden. My world was suspended as I shared these intimate moments with her. Her world—set apart from my twenty-first century life of e-mail, iPods, and cell phones. Only the metronomelike click of the clock and the periodic chime of the bell marked time.

Eventually I needed to use the outhouse. I pulled on my jacket and gloves and faced the darkness with Rita's flashlight. The shack was located about twenty feet from the house. Baring my bottom over the wooden hole was chilly. Think ice cubes and glaciers and you'll understand the experience.

Back inside, I washed my hands with a bar of soap in a basin of warm water near the stove. Grandmother handed me a mug of hot tea and Rita told me that it was time to do another cervix check. Ann was now six centimeters.

Rita rechecked and said, "The head is applied to the cervix. Let's break her bag of waters." Ann positioned herself over the plastic sheet and towels. After gloving, I carefully peeled the paper from the crochet-like plastic hook and jabbed it through the amniotic sack. Rita noted the time on Ann's chart. Her contractions intensified and were stacked back to back; there was some bleeding. The baby's heart tones remained steady and strong. Gradually the contractions spaced out. We settled back into our routine and Rita returned to the kitchen, then carried in a ceramic basin filled with warm water. She showed me how to apply warm compresses to Ann's perineum to help to soften and stretch her skin.

As I supported Ann, helping her find a comfortable position, applying the warm cloths to her bottom, and handing her a glass of juice, I reflected on how much I had learned about labor from the midwives. Unlike many doctors, they did not appear at the end just in time to catch the baby. Instead they labored with the patients, recommending changes of position, counseling them on how to breathe through contractions with gentle supportive coaching, helping the woman's body open for the birth.

Intense contractions were coming every two minutes now; Ann was too engrossed in the labor to talk. Rita reappeared with the sound of the alarm and instructed me to do another cervical check. Ann was complete—the cervix fully dilated and paper thin.

"Time to push," Rita announced.

Herman came in from the kitchen and checked on his wife.

"Sit behind me like last time?" she asked.

Dressed in his dark trousers and thick socks, Herman climbed onto the bed behind Ann, creating a chair for her to lean against. She pulled hard on her knees and focused all her energy on pushing the baby out between her legs. A low-pitched moan escaped between her lips as she bore down.

After forty-five minutes of pushing the head began to emerge. Rita stood behind me as I caught the baby with my left hand and controlled the speed of the head's exit with my right. I marveled as the body miraculously turned, the top shoulder emerging perpendicular to Ann's legs. With gentle pressure, I lifted the baby's head and the bottom shoulder popped out. The legs slid after. The body was firm and plump. Rita suctioned out the baby's nose and mouth and laid the pink infant on a towel on Ann's abdomen. "No hurry to cut the cord," Rita said.

Herman rubbed his baby with the towel and peered between its legs. "It's a boy!" he said in his deep resonant voice. Grandmother appeared at the bedroom door with a pile of blankets warmed on the stove. Edward wandered in behind her and crawled up on the bed next to his parents, quietly observing the new baby. "Your brother," Herman said.

We assessed the baby, noting his color, activity, facial expression, respirations, and pulse—the APGAR. The score was nine at one minute and nine again at five minutes. When the pulse in the cord stopped, Rita directed me to place two yellow plastic clamps on it. I then handed Herman the scissors, directing him to cut between the clamps. I stepped back as if I had a camera capturing this intimate family moment. In the halo of the oil lamp: a mother, father, and two sons huddled together on a bed in a one-bedroom farmhouse heated by a woodstove during a Minnesota winter. Grandmother looked on, smiling at the continuation of her lineage.

She carried her new grandson into the kitchen to clean and dress him. The ritual dress of a newborn was a cloth diaper, navy blue or dark green dress, and two swaddling blankets.

"Time to check the placenta," Rita said.

The cord released with a gentle tug. I placed the bloody placenta into a plastic ice cream pail and massaged the uterus as it clamped down. Later Herman would bury the placenta.

Rita inspected and found a tear at the bottom of Ann's perineum that she instructed me to repair. She positioned Herman behind me to hold the oil lamp. At this point I had repaired half a dozen tears and felt confident in my technique, but it was a new experience to sew under the glow of an oil lamp.

When I was finished, Herman helped me move Ann and we stretched fresh sheets on the mattress. Ann climbed back under the patchwork quilt and Grandmother handed her the swaddled baby. Rita and I lingered for another hour: helping the baby latch on to Ann's breast, completing paperwork, checking to make sure that Ann was not bleeding. I examined the baby on the bed under Edward's wide-eyed gaze. Reluctantly, I handed the baby back to Ann, patting him one more time to say goodbye.

As we drove down the lane, the brocade sky, a composite of tangerine and watermelon streaked with silver, announced the imminent arrival of the sun. Corn stalks still holding the husks of the ears dotted the fields that stretched to the horizon. The rolling cropland was occasionally interrupted by a small stand of trees that protected a house, barn, and a family. A new day, another "all-nighter," and I wasn't even tired.

A shorter version of this story was published in *Family Medicine* 40.2 (2008): 91–92.

Lost On Call

ANN NEUSER LEDERER

I was on call, and tense. Newly employed as a visiting nurse
on the edges of Appalachia, I had recently moved to this place
from a large rust belt city hundreds of miles to the north.
Our territory extended down to the river cliffs,
and outward through patchworks of farms.
I didn't know it very well, especially in the dark.

It was a weeknight. I was tired from the day's work.
The beeper jolted me awake.
I fumbled into my clothes, neatly folded nearby, awaiting.
I was called out to a place I had never been, on the edge of the county,
to a death of a patient I had never known.
It was the middle of the night. There were no lights anywhere.
I peered at the directions written on the paper.

Ever so slowly I made my way down the winding tree-lined lane.
It was one of those roads with steep drops on both sides and no shoulders.
Only the halo ahead, created by the headlights,
hinted which way the next curve might lead.
As I turned a bend, I spotted from the corner of my eye an odd red glow,
low to the ground, seemingly coming out of nowhere.
Slowly, I realized it was a pile of something smoldering.
I did not know anything about field fires then.

Wondering, tempted to imagine, I forced myself to attend to the task at hand.
I could not find the turn-in for the house. I must have passed it, so I backtracked,
tried again, a little scared. A full moon rose over the bare tree limbs,
soothing me with its steady presence. I followed a twisty road up a hill.
Far to the back of a farm, a trailer was parked. This was the place.
They sat, awaiting my knock.

They had no running water. The corpse had soiled himself,
maybe a good while before dying. They wanted him clean for the mortician.
They brought a bucket and I tried my best.
Fresh diaper, and shirt, buttoned to the neck. Hair brushed. Mouth closed.
Ready.
Now, the red glow in the dark field, the white moon above,
lighting the road up the hill are permanent reminders of potential surprises,
against the nights of dread.

Spring and All, Revisited
—after William Carlos Williams

RICHARD M. BERLIN

By the road home from the general hospital
under the surge of the pink
towering clouds drifted from the
southwest—a warm wind. Beyond, the
edge of a mountain pond, redwings
on bulrush calling out their claims,

circle of black water
the veil of thin ice, receding

All along the road, the same reddish
purplish, forked, upstanding twiggy
stuff of bushes you saw years ago

Damp and buzzing, spirited
spring awakens—

Pickerel feed in the shallows,
skunk cabbage on the shore emerges
brownish-purple and mottled-green,
shell-like and hot
around the knob of tiny flowers,
above them, a great blue
heron, alert, waiting

And I think of you, Doc Williams
stopping by the road to the contagious
hospital that morning, standing in a
cold Jersey wind
before the rush of nurses in starched

uniforms and white-winged
caps, your patients with diseases
I'll never see, like the ferocious
little girl with diphtheria in "The Use of Force"

Right now I'm a hundred and fifty
miles from the waste of your broad
muddy fields, the end
of a day with dementia and AIDS,
headed home to redefine
the objects in my world—

raw knuckles of red
rhubarb breaking the earth's clay crust,
sawed-off apple limbs expecting fire,
sticky-swollen horse chestnut buds,
tips sharpened to stingers aimed at the sky,
all around, the grass a rumor of green

Robotic Docs: Excerpts from Dick Gordon's
The Story, *National Public Radio*

DICK GORDON

"That's your doctor up there," the nurse explains pointing to the small camera in the corner of the hospital room in Sioux Center, Iowa. Eighty-nine year old William Sneller lies in his hospital bed, having suffered another heart attack. Because Sioux Center participates in the eICU (electronic-intensive care unit), Mr. Sneller can stay put. He won't have to travel the seventy miles by ambulance to Sioux Falls to receive the intensive care he needs.

His son waves to the camera.

A voice responds, "I see you there."

"Your doctor's talking to you," the nurse says. "A few patients have thought it was God."

Watching them is an "intensivist," a doctor who specializes in caring for critically ill patients in the ICU. Using video cameras and monitors connected by fiber-optic lines, an intensivist physician and one or two nurses in one location are able to care for patients in multiple locations. Think about how air traffic controllers and onboard technology for pilots keeps fliers safe, and you'll understand how an eICU team keeps patients safe in a variety of smaller hospitals. The eICU team monitors dozens of hospitalized patients located long distances away, using computers and cameras.

Today's technology gives the intensivist team all they need. With the electronic medical record, they can read notes written by the nurses and doctors in the community hospital and write orders that can be carried out immediately. The camera resolution allows the intensivist to examine a skin lesion or check pupil reactions. Blood pressure, respirations, and heart tracings can be watched simultaneously. Conversations are abbreviated because the intensivist team can see what is happening with the patient and the nurse caring for him.

Studies show that this model of care can reduce ICU mortality by 25 percent and save costs. The keys are constant surveillance, providing the patient with immediate intensivist access, and arming the intensivist with the patient information needed to make the right decisions, quickly.[1] However, this is an additional expense for the community hospital that cannot always be passed on to the patient's insurance. Physicians caring from afar may be less likely to consider the financial impact on the patient's bill or the community hospital's bottom line.[2] The good news is that telemedicine can support the community hospital and its team of doctors and nurses in providing high-quality and up-to-date care and minimize the need to hire more specialists, rack up transportation costs, and delay needed care.[3]

Mr. Sneller is happy to stay put. He's lived in Sioux Center most of his life. He knows and trusts the nurses here. His children who work in town can stop by during their lunch hours and after work; they don't need to take time off work. Of course, if Mr. Sneller did not have the eICU option, he could have refused the transfer to Sioux Falls and accepted the fact that this was probably the end of his long and happy life. Right now, Mr. Sneller feels lucky to have another option.

Notes

1. eICU Integrated Healthcare Solution for Critical Care, 13 March 2008 <http://www.visicu. com/products/index.html>.

2. Ibid.

3. Fourth Annual AAMC Physician Workforce Research conference April 30–May 2, 2008. Hyatt Regency, Crystal City VA. New Models of Care and Workforce Implications.

Excerpted with permission, broadcast 16 October 2007. Available at <http://thestory.org/archive/ the_story_363_Robotic_Docs.mp3/view>.

A Vow of Connectedness: Views from the Road to Beaver's Farm

DAVID LOXTERKAMP

We are leaving town on Marsh Road. In the driver's seat of the Toyota pickup is my friend Michael Simon. Today we are searching for a Mother's Day gift for my wife, Lindsay, but our journey is also a gift between friends.

The road winds west by Dyer's Woodworking Shop and its lawn circus of windmills, wishing wells, weather vanes, lighthouses, and flagpoles. We pass by shacks and trailers, the Marsh Road Group Home, and the homestead of Joseph Miller, our community's founder. A right fork onto Poor's Mill Road draws us to the floor of the Passagassawakeag River Valley.

Here the abandoned triple-decker chicken barns, the unpainted farmhouses, and collapsed machine sheds all whisper the decline of a flourishing farm economy. Six miles from town, we cross the river Passy, then overtake it again on our meander to Morrill Village at the nine-mile mark. This small cluster of buildings boasts the Morrill Baptist Church, the elegant iron gates of Morrill Cemetery overlooking Smith's Millpond, and the Morrill General Store. Left on Berry Road and two miles beyond, we finally arrive at Beaver Simmons's farm, a dairy operation on the ridge of Morey Hill that he purchased in 1973.

On this rise, Beaver raised six children, established a small lumber mill, increased his pastures, built two log cabins, and maintained sixty head of dairy cattle before passing the reins to his sons. My practice partner, Dr. Tim Hughes, once asked Beaver how he, as a city boy from New York, ever ended up in a milking barn. He replied that it was the scent of the stalls that hooked him, a mixture of manure and silage, limestone, and the breath of cows.

I have known Beaver for a dozen years. He is a member of my parish, a patient in our practice, the host of our son's summer camp excursions, and a grandfather figure for my daughter, who helps with the summer milking. His daughter-in-law once worked in our medical office. He and Dr. Hughes forged their friendship years ago in Tim's two-man racing shell. One of Beaver's sons married the next-door neighbor (she had been among my children's favorite babysitters).

Momentarily we spot Beaver, warm to his boyish smile, and shake his rough-hewn hand, then follow him to the manure pit behind the barn. This concrete basin, fifty feet square by eight feet deep, was built with federal dollars to curtail fecal runoff into Smith's Millpond Bog lying directly below. The basin is filled from the bottom up by a pump from the barn, so that the most thoroughly composted manure rises and crusts at the surface. I have come to buy some of this worm-wealthy manure because my wife is a gardener, and I know her needs. We skim shovelfuls of this desiccated "black gold" into feed bags and load them on the pickup. After hoisting the last bag, Michael fancies taking a shortcut across the manure pile. It trembles ominously beneath his weight, then buckles. But he is in luck: I am within arm's length and provide the leverage to wriggle him free.

Before leaving, Beaver invites us to the log cabin he fashioned entirely by hand. We talk of pioneers and applejack, then Beaver drives us back up the meadow along a path lost in waves of alfalfa. Suddenly the truck stalls, and Michael and I tumble out to push as tires whir and slide on the grass-greased slope. At the top, Beaver thanks us for our help. Thank us? As we drive back to Belfast, I ask Michael how I might compensate a man who refuses any payment for his precious manure. With a shrug of the shoulders he replies, "You already have."

CONNECTEDNESS

Sixteen years of practice in Belfast, Maine, has made me a part of the wider community. I am linked to patients' lives by more than the designation as their primary provider. There is a natural logic to it, as obvious and real as the stream that flows from Smith's Millpond Bog to my home at the mouth of Belfast Bay. Together we have learned how waste can both pollute and fertilize the land around us. My patients, in their Yankee bullheadedness and patched-together lives, assure me that I belong here. We—forever denying this fact—seem to need one another.

POLITICS

One can be seduced into politics by the notion that popularity, moral righteousness, and a good grasp of the playing field are a guarantee for success. So, soon after establishing myself in medical practice, I joined the parish council, spoke up at hospital staff meetings, and ran for the school board. Mine was a voice for family practice values. I helped children become more involved in church worship, opposed screening programs that reduced health care to a commodity, and supported neighborhood schools that fostered strong relationships between teachers and the wider community.

In these and other debates, I was frequently on the losing side. You might have thought that medicine—where the patient's struggle against mortality is conceded from the start—would have prepared me for poor outcomes. Even in victory, the politician is left with a compromised and transitory gain. He must cherish the political process more than the final vote—likewise, the doctor's reward, which lies in a love of his or her patients and the provision of good care rather than in any false hope of transforming the misery that parades past his or her door.

CHANGE

Is the family doctor an agent of social or political change? Perhaps some of us will shape and leverage the national debate. More will run for elected office in our home state or municipality. The rest will do their part by maintaining the connections that are severed in patients' lives during the course of their disease, despair, addiction, or aging. For them, the doctor holds the flicker of hope, the reassuring hand, a mirror of their self-worth, and sense of dignity. Through our own lives, we model the possibility of change.

I have saved only a few of my patients. I have seen alcoholics give up the bottle, wives flee the battering hand, the morbidly obese shed an elephant riding on their backs. But most of what the doctor accomplishes is infinitesimally small, barely a quiver, broad and trickling like the St. John's River for those who are succored in the watershed of our care. We are stewards of a human ecology. Our practices are strengthened by diversity, interdependence, and the desire for our mutual long-term survival. We are caretakers of what Robert Putnam calls "social capital."

The wife of a patient of mine, home dying of lung cancer, recently said to me, "Dr. Loxterkamp, I just feel better knowing that you drive by my house every morning."

A child in church, whose cerebral palsy limits her to a space-age motility device, often hovers at my pew. At first I tried to ignore her, disturbed as I was by her jerking and drooling and those penetrating eyes. I feared that any attention might lodge her there permanently. But, once I touched her outstretched finger, she moved on, satisfied by the meeting of our fingers. Now others safely do the same.

I recently attended the coroner's case of a girl I had delivered eight years prior. She had darted into the path of an oncoming car and died, as I soon discovered, instantly of a broken neck. When I called her father with my merciful news, he sounded grateful. But there was one favor he now dared to ask of me: since I had been there for her birth, been there at her death, would I honor them by being there, too, at their daughter's funeral?

THE PRACTICE

The only place a family doctor—this family doctor—can create lasting change is in his own backyard. Over the years I have exercised this prerogative just four times. Nine years ago my partner and I provided each other with a year's sabbatical. After our reunion, we instituted the Thursday Morning Meeting, wherein providers gather for an hour each week to examine the enemy within. Earlier this year, we banned pharmaceutical representatives and their samples from our office. Shortly thereafter, I set a date for my retirement ten years hence (at age fifty-seven) when I shall remove the mantel of full-time physician.

These changes were the gift of sight. One year's leave of absence taught me that practice is a privilege, the practitioner a nonessential cog in its continuance. Within the support group, I began to articulate, for the first time among peers, the sense of insecurity, blurred boundaries, fallibility, and an unmitigated need for forgiveness that we all share. Rejecting drug samples and industry propaganda forced us to acknowledge the barriers to free and informed choice that we ourselves had erected. And, setting the date of my retirement was a cock paid to my mortality and a first step toward helping younger colleagues—and my children—transition to the helm.

During my tenure in Belfast, I have witnessed (and been party to) the drama of doctors who could not retire and instead squandered their reputations on vestiges of power and self-purpose. I have known peers (and their temptation) to satisfy personal needs at the expense of their patients. I have watched my medical community isolate itself from the sources of feedback and support that I credit with my own survival.

PROFESSIONALISM

The family doctor is a hybrid in the field of medicine. We perform the generalist's role with specialists' ambitions. We are amateurs (from the Latin *amator*) who love our labor and shoot more from the hip than from the sights of expert opinion. We still consider medicine a vocation, or calling, and thus remain open to duty that lies beyond the roles for which we're prepared. And, we remember that professionals are those who profess something publicly about what they believe.

I have listened to the professions of Trappist monks at New Melleray, Gethsemani, and New Clairvaux abbeys. Not only do they commit themselves to the religious life (in the vows of poverty, chastity, and obedience) but pledge to live in one place (the vow of stability) in order that grace, working through community, may move them (by a conversion of manners) closer to God.

Family doctors, too, understand that our high incomes distort our perceptions of the poor; money tests our personal values and stands between patients and their access to medical care. Chastity reminds us to be respectful of the intimacies we guard and faithful to those who are marginalized by the loss of insurance or physical well-being. We remain obedient to a higher authority—the precepts of science and a moral conduct befitting our profession. We realize that patient care is not portable and that the doctor who lives among his mistakes and prejudices becomes a healthier person less prone to severity in the judgment of patients or peers. Lastly, family doctors are inevitably changed by the patients they serve. The merely responsible physician, tempered by mercy and groomed by grace, adds to the stock of moral credibility that has sustained our profession over the millennia.

What I am trying to describe is a doctor who is more than the sum of his or her parts, more than a tally of screening tests and minor procedures and patient encounters scored over the course of a career. We might more easily see that a rabbi or minister is not only master of ceremonies but a person praised as a man of God. We know that a teacher is more than a conveyor of facts and proctor of exams but someone dedicated to the channeling of curiosity in the pursuit of truth. So, too, family doctors, who through the blur of ICD-9 and CPT codes will finally rest in those relationships that define and sustain their work.

WHAT ARE COWS FOR?

Six years ago, Dr. Tim Hughes took time off again to enroll as an extern with *Salt Magazine*. For his journalism project, he focused on the growing debate over bovine synthetic somatostatin (BST). Under what conditions—with what labels or restrictions—would the state allow BST to enter the state's milk supply? Monsanto Corporation had spent a quarter billion dollars developing and marketing Posilac, a biologically engineered hormone that had been shown to increase milk production by 10 percent when injected into cows. Despite safety endorsements from nearly every major medical, nutritional, and scientific group—and finally, in 1993, FDA approval—politicians, consumers, and the state's six hundred dairy farmers were divided on its risks and benefits.

For his sources, Tim interviewed two dairy farmers who had given opposing testimony to a state legislative subcommittee. He traveled to Cornell University to speak with the original investigator and national spokesperson for BST, Professor Dale Bauman. Dr. Bauman was understandably convinced of the safety and societal need of BST: "When you do the population curve and project it out . . . then all the food needed in the world for the next forty years is equal to the amount that was previously produced in the history of humankind. This ability to make gains in the productivity of animal and plant agriculture is really important in the long term [and] productivity is what BST is all about."
Stewart Smith, a former state commissioner of agriculture and professor of sustainable agriculture at the University of Maine, offered a tempering view. He saw a relationship between farmers' enthusiasm for biotechnological solutions (in contrast to management-intensive practices) and the structure and funding of agricultural research. He lamented farming's shrinking role in the food sector, from 41 percent in 1910 to 9 percent in 1990. The use of BST, he felt certain, would transfer even more cash from the farmer to Monsanto. He asked why the dairy industry needed more productivity when there has long been a milk surplus. BST in the marketplace would reduce the need for dairy cows and, consequently, the number of farmers to tend them. Is it worth asking, he wonders, if farming itself is a social good?

Beaver Simmons is the embodiment of Smith's philosophical argument against BST. He considers any potential health risk unacceptable for his cows. "As far as I'm concerned, it's abusive. And what right do I have to abuse my cows?" Beaver is headstrong in his distrust of chemical companies and believes that the greatest adverse effect of BST is to turn cows into machines.

Beaver farms the way I would like my son and daughter to live—with passion, respect, and gratitude. He is committed to his land and livestock and adheres to a high (albeit unspoken) moral code. The lowing of the milk barn is his calling; its sweet scent his ample reward. He grasps the rule of interdependence between the husbandman and his herd.

The bond between family practice and rural America goes deeper than a historical regard for the cradle of general practice. It cannot be explained by the fact that many of our leaders were raised on agrarian values. I can tell you that it is easier to be a family doctor and to feel a sense of connection and interdependence in a small community than it is in a large one—just as it is easier to sustain one's religion in a monastery than in a mall. The conditions are ripe for the receptive mind.

While the specialties add to the clinical knowledge base and perfect our techniques, family practice quietly concerns itself with improving the doctor. We, like the evangelist Matthew, take seriously Jesus' rebuke to the Pharisees, "Go and learn the meaning of the words: mercy is what pleases me, not sacrifice." We ruminate on the question Tim Hughes forks at our feet, "What are cows for?"

The family doctor is rarely an agent of meteoric change. But, every day and closer to the earth, we are its vehicle and eyewitness. Doctors who remain deeply connected to their patients will know this privilege, as will those of us who retain the capacity to listen, touch, and tether ourselves to the wounds of others. In modest ways, we accomplish the utterly profound, long before the prescription is filled or the blood test is taken. We profit by the patients' periodic return and by the mutual exchange of friendship, intimacy, and trust.

What are cows for? To the bioengineer and corporate manager, they are machines; they are units of production. But, to those who have experienced "farming itself as an end, the stewardship and husbanding of the land, the plants, and the animals," as Dr. Hughes observes, " . . . a cow is, above all else, a living thing to be respected if she is to enrich our own life." He might have said also that cows can bring us joy and beauty, provide companionship, and inspire the next generation of farmers to love and care for them. They can sustain a small business and livelihood that relies on sustainable relationships with crops, animals, and the earth and on the natural intersection between life and death.

Clearly, my mind has wandered to the broader question: what are patients for and by extension the family doctors and their technologies? It is the most unsettled and unsettling of questions. It rises from a vow of connectedness and is the sentinel for those of us who seek change—in our patients and in ourselves—through the exercise of our art.

This essay was published in *Family Medicine* 33.4 (2001): 244–47.

Whom We Serve

Whom We Serve—Synopsis

THERESE ZINK AND TARA FRERKS

"The calls and visits blindside you. You will prepare and prepare, and you will never be prepared," writes Michael Perry, nurse, firefighter, and emergency medical responder. For the men and women like Michael, who are called to a crash on a country road or to a farmhouse in the middle of the night, to the nurses and physicians at the hospital who receive his patients, there are always surprises. The geography isolates you, you confront the limits of your knowledge and your resources, even with today's technology. You learn to work with what you have and discover the confidence and creativity it takes to "go it alone." This same pioneering spirit and desire for autonomy carried settlers into the heartland and west. Today new Americans, documented and undocumented, like Dr. Ercole's Rosa respond to the same yearning and do what they have to do to pursue a better life: *No hay las mismas oportunidades en México para mis hijos como las que hay aquí.* (There are not the same opportunities in Mexico for my children as they would have here.) Others, originally from Africa and Asia and invited by local churches, make new homes in small towns across the United States. These new Americans do jobs that few U.S. citizens want to do, working in meat-packing and food-processing plants and harvesting crops. As a result, the faces in rural America are increasingly diverse.

Rural counties, especially those located adjacent to metropolitan areas have seen population growth. Challenges arrive along with these new Americans: How do two or three different cultures live together? How does a small clinic with limited resources accommodate different languages and different understandings about health and healing? The diabetic diet looks different from a Mexican diet where beans and rice are staples and different from the farmer who wants his meat and potatoes. Some workers arrive without family, leaving their wives and children back home for the season or several years. Problems such as alcohol abuse, sex trafficking, and violence often accompany this disconnected lifestyle.

Nestled into the rural landscape are populations like the Amish who seek a place where they can live their traditional family values. Although it may be easier to achieve this in rural America, the longing for small communities to hold fast to old-fashioned values may be the wishful fantasies of nostalgic Americans. The realities are, as indicated by the headlines in newspapers across rural America, that even the heartland confronts the same moral and cultural dilemmas that plague the big cities. There is AIDS (Dr. Gutterman's "Hanging On for Your Life") and the stigma associated with the diagnosis, especially in a small community where one's business is not so private.

Dr. Brodt recounts the shooting that occurred in the high school on the Indian reservation near his childhood home and the emotional and professional challenges of responding. These were not just trauma patients with gunshot wounds, for "I played basketball with their brothers, knew their faces from powwows." New and old societal challenges face rural providers. Gangs have invaded some rural communities, demanding new skills for law enforcement and schools. Alcohol abuse and driving while intoxicated, especially for teens and young adults, because there just isn't much else to do, continue to demand attention. More recently, methamphetamine produced from anhydrous ammonia (which is also used by farmers for fertilizer) is a menace. Less publicized are the child abuse, sexual assaults, and elder abuse and neglect, which have occurred for decades and continue to occur behind the closed doors of small-town bungalows and farmhouses.

Health care professionals struggle to respond. Despite the fact that everyone knows everybody's business, there is an eerie silence that accompanies certain diagnoses and problems. Rural populations are overall poorer, in worse general health, and less likely to be insured than people in metropolitan areas. Reimbursement may be subject to the dictates of Medicaid or Medicare, when it is available at all. Resources and social support networks, like mental health, are limited.

Mental illness may be better tolerated in smaller communities, as described in Dr. Zink's "Asking the Right Questions." But patients with mental health concerns may also be harder to identify because they may be reticent to fully disclose symptomatic information to their clinician, someone they see also see at church. And then there is the "code of secrecy," not wanting relatives or neighbors to know that they are seeking help "for mental problems." At the same time, rural values such as self-reliance and self-care may delay others in reaching out for help. Old man Geisen, Dot's father, (William Orem's "I Am the Handmaiden of the Lord") was unimpressed with what the big-city clinic had to offer; in fact, he was incensed that Dot was referred there at all. However, Dr. Rosmann's Kent ("Cattleman") clearly benefited from the help of his psychologist. Rural areas suffer from a scarcity of mental health professionals as well as other health care providers like nurses, doctors, and dentists—the distance often limits access. With inadequate staff, professionals face heavy workloads and on-call demands; limited professional networks create a solitariness that engenders loneliness. There is a discomfort that comes with small-town life; it is common to encounter a patient in social settings, blurring professional and personal boundaries.

More than one-fourth of the rural population is over sixty-five, a higher proportion than in metropolitan areas. With an aging population comes the need for a variety of social supports, especially to help them continue to live in their homes. Home health aids like Holly Farris, homecare nurses like Ann Neuser Lederer, physicians like Drs. Stuart and Fleg who make house calls, allow seniors to do what most want to do—stay where they have resided for decades. "I want to garden, I like my things, I like the view out the kitchen window," I've had my own elderly patients tell me. After all, living at home is cheaper than nursing home placement, even with all the social supports. Fleg, Farris, and Lederer capture the delights and headaches encountered with homes visits. One headache is that some services are not covered by insurance, and frugal seniors are often unwilling to pay for them. As their doctor, you straddle between allowing grandma to stay home and worrying about her safety.

There are no easy answers when Depression-era frugality and life savings meet pricey health care. The family home may be willed to the children, but the realities of caring for ailing relatives are often too much for a generation of adult children who are pulled in many directions and often live a plane trip away. Both adults need to work to make ends meet, farming hardly supports you anymore, and mother rarely has the luxury of staying home with the kids. Kids have scheduled lives today and need to be shuttled between activities. How can the adult children possibly find time to care for their frail and often demented parents? County social supports struggle to meet the challenges of geography and the strained budgets that are thin because taxpayers want to keep the government out of their lives.

Our high-tech health care system allows us to do almost anything but racks up the costs exponentially. There are some tough choices. Today's practitioners will not diagnose diphtheria, but they are faced with AIDS, dementia, and the challenges of when to prolong life, what interventions to recommend, and how to end the treatments provided when those treatments are no longer improving a patient's ability to enjoy life. Dr. Kollisch eloquently describes the challenges Elwin faced when the burdens of "no salt, no straining, no riding the John Deere by myself anymore" make the days less bearable ("Good Will"). Other selections in other sections grapple with these challenges. Dr. Vainio describes his struggle with knowing when to quit ("Mashkikiwinini: Thanking Sylvester for His Unconditional Smile"), asking when does technology enhance or detract from the quality of a patient's life. Some families avoid these choices, and all involved suffer the consequences (Therese Zink's "Everyone Did Their Part, But"). Other families, like Dr. McRay's, help their loved one come to terms with the illness and discover that there are choices that can be made ("Three Days Changed My Grandfather's Life"). Despite the existence of advanced directives, physicians forget to tell patients about them, and thorough discussions about the pros and cons of proceeding with a technology that will prolong life are rare. Would Elwin have been better off without the valve replacement? Would McRay's grandfather have said no to dialysis if he understood that there was a choice? For Mr. Gains ("Everyone Did Their Part, But"), repairing the hip fracture appeared to be the right option if he was to ambulate again. Technology prolongs life and often provides treasured months and years for some, but the benefits are less clear for others. All in all, the challenges of caring for the citizens of rural America today are abundant, as are the gifts.

Pursuing the American Dream:
The Human Face of Immigration

CESAR EMILIO ERCOLE

As I picked up my morning fruit from the doctors' lounge, the day's newspaper headline jumped out: "Illegal Immigrant Kills Passenger and Injures Daughter in Car Crash." The driver, Rosa Hernandez, was a patient I had seen in the clinic days earlier. She was now the unofficial poster child for advocates of tighter borders and better background checks in order to prevent "those people from coming here."

As part of my third year of medical school, I was spending nine months in the small midwestern town where Rosa was living. Born in Detroit, Michigan, I had learned Spanish at an early age from my parents who grew up in Argentina. The clinic and hospital to which I was assigned served a large Spanish-speaking population, many of whom were undocumented. My preceptor, Dr. Madison, is fluent in Spanish and has a reputation for treating all and is willing to manage separate charts—one with the real and one with the borrowed names and birthdates.

Like many midwestern communities that were settled by Scandinavian and German immigrants, this community was adjusting to a growing Latino population, many of whom were employed by the local meat-processing plants. Immigrations and Customs Enforcement agents recently descended on our town, claiming they were looking for illegal immigrants with criminal backgrounds. Many people didn't believe them, so they did not go to work and kept their children home from school. One patient told me that she hid a frightened friend in her attic for two days. Few Latinos, regardless of status, frequented the local stores. We had five clinic cancellations.

I met Rosa, a shy thirty-three-year old, two days before her accident. She sat in the exam room with her shoulders tense and legs crossed waiting for her annual physical. She made only intermittent eye contact when I first asked how she had obtained her borrowed name. After reassurances about my sincerity, she appeared to relax. Her eyes beamed intensely as she described how she had methodically saved money in Mexico and then twelve years ago walked across the border to California and bought her social security number for $1,500.

She explained, *No hay buen trabajo en México. Es muy difficile.* (There are no good jobs in Mexico. It is very difficult.) She had worked under the assumed identity, choosing to delay marriage and children until a few years ago when she had laid aside enough savings and had secured a stable job. Now she had a husband and a twenty-two-month-old daughter.

I asked her about returning to Mexico.

She vehemently shook her head. *No hay las mismas oportunidades en México para mis hijos como las que hay aquí.* (There are not the same opportunities in Mexico for my children as they would have here.) Unlike some of the other undocumented patients, she wanted to establish roots here. Her sister was in the process of getting her citizenship, and Rosa hoped that once her sister was a U.S. citizen, then she could secure her own citizenship.

We discussed the more reactionary views some Americans held of the Hispanic/Latino population. *Es muy triste,* she said. "The media and people tend to focus on those that are doing bad things—the gangs, the drug dealers. They don't tell the stories of the hard workers, those who give back to the community."

Undocumented patients do not see their illegal immigration as anything malicious. While it includes establishing a false identity and obtaining welfare, these actions are seen as necessary in order to obtain a better life. *No hay las mismas oportunidades en México.*

Two days later, Rosa was admitted to the hospital after smashing her pickup into a storefront at the local mall. The nursing staff had read the front-page story. Many expressed concern for Rosa's daughter and her passenger; a few judged her. One said, "She should get life in jail for her irresponsibility."

During our brief encounter, I had come to know Rosa as a kind and industrious person. When I pulled up her labs on the computer and saw that her tox screen showed a blood alcohol level twice the legal limit, I was disappointed. I had such hope for Rosa. Now, I could only imagine the impending consequences.

Three friends surrounded Rosa in her hospital room, as she blankly stared out the window, a much sadder version of the woman I had met only days before. She had just learned that her companion in the front seat had died. Her friends asked questions for her: When would Rosa be discharged? When could she see her daughter?

"I'll check," I said, happy to do something useful. Over in the pediatric ward, Rosa's daughter, barely two, sat quietly in her bed. Rosa's husband, also Mexican, was helping his daughter with her breakfast. Concerned for his wife, he asked when she would be allowed to see their daughter. I called Dr. Madison who arranged for Rosa to visit her daughter and husband before we discharged her home.

A few days later Rosa had a follow-up appointment at the clinic to remove her stitches. She remained apathetic and despondent. Her main concern was getting an excuse for having missed work due to the accident. It was evident she did not grasp the gravity of what had happened and how it would change her life. I warned Dr. Madison about Rosa's naïveté before he joined us. Gently he spoke with her in Spanish about what might happen.

"Qué?" she asked.

"You will probably get arrested and charged because of your friend's death, the alcohol, and property damage," he explained.

That evening the police did arrest Rosa. She was charged with seven felonies, including vehicular homicide, and later was indicted on two counts of fraud for obtaining welfare under a false name. Now Rosa is viewed as one of "those people."

"You hear the news?" my neighbor asked as we brought our trash to the curb. "One of those welfare defrauders stole my tax dollars to buy a pickup truck, then in a drunken escapade . . . crashed it."

As Rosa sat in jail, the local paper started using her real name, and citizens debated the pros and cons of illegal immigration on message boards and in public forums. Some condone the false identities and false welfare claims—their only perceived option for pursuing the American dream. The other options are long and arduous. A few proclaim (inadvertently) their bigotry and ignorance. The majority tries to add some clarity and understanding to a very difficult issue. The meat-packing plants depend on undocumented workers.

The other day I performed a physical on Maria Lopez who told me about her recent journey across the Mexican border, another worker to fill the void of those who are gone.

Postscript: Rosa's daughter was seen in clinic for her two-year well-child visit. She was accompanied by her aunt who is fluent in English. Under home environment it was noted: "Mom in jail, dad gone."

This piece was published in the February 2009 issue of *Minnesota Medicine*.

Cord

HOLLY FARRIS

Some definitions for "cord" from an old dictionary of mine:
1: strings consisting of several strands woven or twisted together
2: a moral, spiritual, or emotional bond
4: a unit of wood cut for fuel

I see in today's midweek edition of the newspaper that they buried her on Tuesday. I'm disappointed, but not about missing the funeral or even that it came so soon. It's that the Wednesday paper always showers bright, slick, advertising flyers as soon as I touch it, leaving me nothing but sooty obits.

"I'm gonna pee," she had said, her first words to me, the Sunday nurse. A warning would have been nice, especially since I had sat, all white and comforting, for an entire morning beside her wheelchair. She was braked next to her smoky egg-and-milk splashed refrigerator. Before I could lift her to the portable toilet, she'd filled my left white shoe with yellow. Where her cotton nightgown rode up, I saw bones looking like they bloomed along their shafts, enlarged and poking out, lively inside papery skin wrapping. "You smoke?" she said, the second thing. "Nah," she answered herself, "I know from your smell." She was blind, had been before the wheelchair. She couldn't see the family's instructions, her own signature, not to resuscitate if the rescue squad came. The paper was glued, curling and threatening as her old, mean fingernails, right to the face of the refrigerator.

"Got to get dressed for church," she spouted and began digging through the topmost buttonhole into her pitiful gray chest. "You're home from church," I said, sounding too final about where she hadn't been seen for years, but I was grateful that pink blood, sap of the living, leaked out of her wrecked carcass. Then she was on to her naked scalp, scratching close to bald eyebrow ghosts, what burnt-out charcoal remained of her eyes.

"Look," I nearly shouted, stern before I thought how stupid it was to say it. "Look at your nice hair." I picked up her dead starfish hand, stroking it up and down the thick braid I wore over my left shoulder. Freeing the end of the braid's warm rope from its elastic tie, I let strands unravel, curl and stack on her stained nightgown. Hair heaped like cordwood, tangled like last year's twigs snapped for kindling. Her knobby fingers measured the width of strands, plentitude and protection she couldn't hoard against the approaching chill. Weeks ago, her family had pitched the last of her firewood into their pickup held together with baling twine, desperate to heat themselves at her wake.

"See my nice hair?" she had said to the evening nurse when she stepped though the doorway to replace me, within the same half hour our patient died. "You smoke?"

This piece was published in Farris's collection of short fiction, *Lockjaw Collected Appalachian Stories* (Gival Press, 2007).

Good Will

DONALD KOLLISCH

"Like a sponge," Elwin was thinking, sitting in his father's old chair. "The doctor said my lungs are filled up like a sponge that they need to wring out." He pictured a large sponge—the kind his father used to use to wipe down the horses after a full day's work, knobby and heavy and dripping in his hands. Elwin held the image in his mind as he tried to clear his laboring lungs. Some sections were softer and more supple; others were stiff and scarred. Water was stuck in the stiffer cavities so he wasn't able to squeeze it out. That was what made his breathing fast and shallow—the way it had been ever since he'd come in from moving the John Deere into the barn. Now he was sitting at the kitchen table in a sweat.

He heard Doris on the phone saying, "Doctor, I'm bringing Elwin in again. He can't breathe—the valve must be stuck again. I'm bringing him straight to the hospital. Can you get them ready? Jesus, Doctor, it's awful bad this time."

She had found him wheezing in the kitchen and had fixed him with a glare. "You foolish old son of a dog, you've done it again, haven't you? Gone and cut hay when the boys were out just to prove you could do it, just to prove something. Sweet Jesus, when are you going to learn?"

As she half-carried him to the pickup, he remembered how light baby Johnny had been when they'd had to rush him to the hospital for the meningitis. Now, fifty years later, as Doris was carrying Elwin to the same place, he made himself as light as he could so as not to be too hard on her.

The nurses met them at the emergency room ramp with a wheelchair and had an intravenous tube into him in seconds. They gave him a shot of the water medicine right away, too, just like the last time. Elwin pictured his lungs compacting like a cider press as he pushed out each hard breath. He pushed the fluid down through himself and out the tube that they'd slid into his long, curved penis, which hadn't seemed to shrink with age like the rest of him. His urine collected in a plastic bag hooked to the side rail, almost colorless, as they wheeled him to the X-ray machine and then hooked him up to the EKG machine.

"Yup, Elwin, it's the same thing," the doctor said as he scanned the results. "Looks like it's that valve again. I can hear the murmur louder than hell. Any pain this time? I know you go and work on that damn tractor and strain your heart. The valve is too tight and then the heart works too hard and can't push the blood through hard enough, and your lungs fill right up with fluid, and here you are again." He told Elwin about the sponge again, and Elwin did all he could to help squeeze.

Then there was an echo test. Elwin could see his heart pumping on the screen like a cartoon in yellow and green, with thumps and whistles coming out of the speaker. Polly, the echo technician, was daughter to Doris's niece and said that it looked to her like the valve was just as tight as before but no tighter, and that the heart muscle was somewhat weak but still pumping. But she was only the technician, she added. The heart specialist would have to look the next day at the tape she'd produced of the test to make the reading official.

Elwin had gotten to know all of the hospital staff by now. He tried to help each one of them make their jobs less unpleasant; he knew that the nurses and aides were the important ones in the hospital, the ones who—if they liked him—could get him home to his John Deere faster. He was always ready for his pills, ready when they came to change the bed, ready for the walks down the hallway. He pictured his insides and made sure his bowels worked after the change of shift so the night nurse would leave happy. Then Janice, the day nurse, would be cheerful and humming as she helped him into the bathroom and wiped his bottom—just as, he figured, she wiped her son's bottom and hummed before leaving for work.

When his hand slipped and he spilled the water in the blue plastic pitcher that sat by his bed, he got Doris to clean it up so the aides wouldn't hold it against him and tell the doctor that he was still weak and needed to stay in the hospital longer. Doris was used to this and murmured, "You silly old man," as she mopped up.

The doctor sat down on the bed the day Elwin was discharged, as he had done at least twice a year for a decade, and went over everything again. "No salt, Elwin. Doris, there is to be no salt for him. You can't make that bacon, he can't have your soup, and you have to tell Johnny not to bring over that smoked ham at the start of hunting season." It was a familiar litany, and Elwin and Doris nodded their understanding. "The nurse will take your catheter out before you go. Remember to take the pills just as I told you."

"Yes, doctor, of course. No salt, no straining, no riding the John Deere by myself anymore. We'll see you in the office next week with that old appointment I've got, you figure?"

"Well, yes, keep that appointment, but there's more this time, something else to talk about." The doctor fingered his graying beard and hesitated. He looked first at Elwin, then at Doris, and then his eyes settled on the clock on the wall. "On that echo test, your valve is getting tighter—getting to be what they call 'critical.' I'm not sure we can keep going from one crisis to the next any more. I think maybe we're going to need to do something. Maybe send you down to the University Hospital for one of the heart surgeons to take a look at you. Maybe replace the valve."

Elwin tried to think about how to help this along. He wanted to get home. "You know me, doctor—I don't want anything special, anything drastic. Just give me medicine and get me home. You know me, doctor." The argument didn't sound even to Elwin's own ears quite strong enough to change the doctor's mind, but the doctor sighed and nodded and signed the order sheet in the chart. "Okay, Elwin, to home with you, but we'll talk again next week. And you be thinking about letting them give you that new valve."

At the doctor's office the next week, Elwin greeted the nurse cheerfully: "Feeling great, Gayle. Doc sure patched me up this time." She wrote "feeling great" in his chart. The doctor mumbled, "Sorry to be running late. Nurse says you're doing good," as he brushed into the examining room. Elwin made it easier. "Like I told Gayle," he spoke up, "I'm feeling fine. Doris is taking care of me just like you said, and Johnny's not letting me mow until you give the word." He watched the doctor carefully to make sure he was shaping his case well. "But last cutting's done anyway, and we're getting ready to get to Florida next month, same as always, get out of the cold. So could you fix me up with some prescriptions, do you think, the way you always do?"

The doctor hesitated, tapped his fingers on the desk, and motioned for Elwin to loosen his shirt. He listened to Elwin's breathing on the back of his chest. His beard brushed Elwin's cheek when he listened in front. "I guess, Elwin, I guess. You really don't want to go down for that new valve, do you?" Elwin looked up at him and shook his head. "I worry about you being down in Florida," the doctor continued, "where they don't know you. I worry that Doris'll bring you to a hospital all worried, the way she gets. And a doctor who doesn't know her and you, doesn't know how these things go with you, will open you right up, and . . . Jesus, Elwin, this isn't a walk in the woods, this surgery, if you know what I mean." Elwin glanced at the door. "A heart attack, a stroke, anything can happen on the table once your valve gets this bad. Can't I send you down to University, so that one of the guys I know can take a look at you?"

Elwin shook his head, with a small grin on his farmer's weathered face, and took the prescriptions the doctor offered him. "I'll see you first thing in the spring, Doc, don't you worry."

Before leaving for Florida, Elwin climbed up onto the John Deere in the shed and sat there for the afternoon, listening to the swallows swooping to and from their nests in the eaves and to the cats chasing mice in the hayloft.

The months of the winter went so fast they were a blur. Afterward, Elwin barely remembered arriving at the trailer park in central Florida. He didn't remember climbing onto the mower to help the park's owners trim the front yard. He didn't remember the pain and breathlessness, the ambulance ride to the unfamiliar hospital, or the tall, stern doctor with the Southern accent telling Doris that surgery was Elwin's only chance. He didn't remember waking up in an intensive care unit with a breathing tube in his throat, unable to move his right arm and leg, unable to ask the nurses what the matter was and how he could help. The doctor had told Doris that Elwin was lucky to have survived the operation at all, but that his new valve was working fine. He said that the stroke was something they had spoken of as a complication when she had signed the papers at the beginning, and that his rehabilitation back up at home would tell the story about how much strength and ability to speak he'd get back.

The first thing Elwin remembered was looking at Doris with tears in his eyes as she tucked a blanket around him in the backseat of Johnny's car for the trip home. "I'm so sorry, my dear old bag of bones, but there isn't anything you can do to help—I know you want to."

On the long ride back home he began to understand. They stopped at their own little hospital as soon as they reached Vermont. The doctor had agreed to meet them there and was waiting for them. His voice cracked when he saw Elwin slumped in the wheelchair, and he carefully unwrapped the blanket to examine him. He took in the flaccid arm, the droop in the face, the pain and fear in Elwin's eyes, and he gently grasped Elwin's arm. "I knew for all of these years how much you've helped me help you. You thought I didn't know, but I did. And now your job is to get as strong as you can. Doris can't take care of you alone, at least for a while, so I've got to put you into the county nursing home to help you recover. They're good down there. You know that. I'll keep you here at the hospital for a couple of days to make the arrangements and then send you down."

Elwin knew then how he could help. After Janice, the day nurse, got him settled in a bed and after Doris left him, he pictured himself on the John Deere, cutting wide swaths in a dense hayfield, the fallen grass lying thick and green and pungent behind him. He reached into the pocket of his barn jacket and pulled out a small hourglass and placed it on the hood of the tractor, where he could watch the sand running down with each pass across the field. And when the last grain ran through, he closed his eyes, the tractor stopped, and he slept.

This piece was first published in *Dartmouth Medicine,* Summer 2000.

Hanging On for Your Life

LORENCE GUTTERMAN

Curled up and bruised, Carter sleeps uncovered on his bed, his sheet rumpled at his feet. Perhaps he shoved it off during a bout of sweats. He has the appearance of being trampled by a bronco. A rodeo rider, he grew up in Minford, a small Ohio farming community.

One of the consulting oncologists from Columbus, Ohio, I travel one hour to this hospital twice a week. I gaze into Carter's room from the hall where I stand and review his chart. This 250-bed hospital, surrounded by cornfields, the Mead Paper Mill, and the Kenworth Truck Company, is a referral center for the nearby small towns. Carter's primary care physician suspects he may have AIDS. I'm not surprised. This is the mid-1990s, and a twenty-seven year old male, like Carter, with high fever, positive blood cultures for *Escherichia coli*, and low blood counts could have AIDS with or without a malignancy.

I knock, enter the room, and introduce myself. Carter rolls over to look at me, a grimace on his face. I step back as the musty air of his room reaches me, reminding me of my high school gym locker room. I brace myself and ask him why he became a rodeo rider.

"My uncle and older brother rode. I wanted to be like 'em. Doc, you want to try it?" He laughs through his obvious misery as he pushes himself into a sitting position, his reedy legs now dangling beneath the flimsy, gray-checkered hospital gown.

"I'm too chicken to sit on a bucking horse," I say and place my chair a safe distance from him. Not so far away to be rude, but I need some space.

"Man, what are ya' afraid of? Thought Docs could do everythin'." His grin changes to a frown as he crosses his legs.

"Believe it or not, doctors get scared." What would my colleagues think of me, admitting vulnerability?

Carter shuts his eyes and rubs them. He clenches his jaw. "Can you give me something for pain? I hurt like hell."

"Of course. I'll talk with your nurse." I quickly leave the room to find his nurse who is counting tablets and putting them into a tiny paper cup. I ask her to increase Carter's dose of morphine. I reenter Carter's room. The odors have not changed. I return to my chair, the cracked vinyl squeaks.

"Hey Doc, ya gonna get me feelin' better?" He has returned to lying down.

"I'll try. Can't promise you though. Could you control the bronco the first time you sat on it?"

He tries to prop himself up on his right elbow. "Doc, ya never can control that animal."

"Kind of like your fever, until I know more about you," I say fidgeting with his chart.

"Those shakes last night, damn! Bounced me around more than any bronc."

"Fever caused your shakes." I stare at the plastic bag filled with clear liquid hanging on a metal pole on the corner of his bed. Its slow drip is hypnotizing, calming. I decide to get to know him before I start quizzing him about risks for AIDS. Taking a sexual history has never been a comfortable task for me. "Where do you do your riding?"

"Lots in southern Ohio. That's where I'm from."

"When did you start riding?"

"In high school." He tells me that he and his buddies skipped class and hung out with older guys. At the rodeo stables he loved feeding and saddling the horses, working with the broncs. He never finished high school, so money has always been a problem. He traveled to ride in rodeos in Kentucky, Indiana, and Michigan. Besides many rough falls, he has had a gouged thigh, a broken arm, and a dislocated shoulder. He rode a saddle bronc, but it was not until his second year that he was able to stay on for the flawless eight seconds. By the third year of riding, he won a couple of contests near Lexington, including his highest prize money of three thousand dollars.

I wonder if the rodeo was his introduction to experiences with other men?

He breaks the silence. "Doc, what's wrong with me?"

"You have an infection."

"What kind?" He pushes himself into a sitting position, quickly covering himself with his gown. "Doc, I hate this gown. Can't keep covered up."

I look away. "Who can we call to bring you pajamas?"

"My wife, Betsy. She's at work. What time is it?"

"Quarter to four," I say looking at my Swiss watch I bought in Grindelwald while on vacation with my wife.

"She cooks in the school cafeteria. Should be here soon."

I stare out his window. The light has moved to a low slant; I am taking too long here. I lead us back to the illness talk. "Bacteria got in your blood, making you sick. Causes the shakes." It's time to wrap this up. "Carter, I need to ask you some questions. Some are personal."

"Like what?"

"About using drugs."

"Drugs?"

"Like pot."

"Sure, I smoked some pot with the guys."

I ask about any other drugs and then about injecting drugs.

"No way," he says and looks at me with surprise.

"Okay." I swallow and ask, "Have you ever had sex with a guy?"

He turns away from me toward the window and shakes his head. "Why do ya' doctors ask so many questions? Can't ya see I feel like shit?"

My anger flares. He's not telling me the truth. I study him. He's lost thirty-five pounds, scrawny as I was as a teen. He smells, the acrid stink of sickness. I reach out to touch his arm, but can't quite do it. "Carter, I want to help you."

"Doc, I'm scared." He faces me again. "Am I going to die?"

At this moment, I can't answer his question. I stand. "Hang in there. You're getting good medicine." My pager beeps. As I move toward the door, Betsy hurries into the room. She breezes past me, not even acknowledging my presence. Her flaxen hair is squeezed into a hairnet, and her steely blue eyes are focused on Carter. She carries a half-empty large Wendy's cup.

"Hey, babe," she says and kisses him on the lips. "You still hurtin'?"

She looks younger than Carter—baby faced, no makeup. Carter introduces her. I shake her hand.

"What do ya think? He's been sick for weeks. He looks awful. Last night at suppertime he hurt a lot. Can ya help him feel better?"

Her rapid-fire manner makes me more aware of my weariness. "I think so." I half lie. Improving the quality of Carter's life may last a few weeks, maybe months. Betsy is asking me for hope. Hope and healing reside somewhere inside my half-truths. But looking at Carter I just can't be optimistic. Still, even if I can't cure Carter's illness, I can ease his pain. I wonder why I do this. I stand there and am glad I'm not the one in the bed, yet. It is always a yet.

Betsy drops her pocketbook and fleece jacket on the other chair. Carter's wince catches my attention as Betsy starts to sit on the bed and reaches over to wipe his forehead with the paper napkin from the Wendy's cup.

"Babe, don't do that," Carter yelps. "Bumpin' the mattress makes me hurt."

"It's gettin' bad when I can't even give ya some lovin'," she fusses and laughs, as she moves off the bed, pushes her purse and jacket on the floor and sits on the chair. "Hon, have they told you anythin'?"

"Not much," Carter says positioning a pillow behind his back.

Betsy's eyes dart from Carter to me. The look changes to a glare. "He's been in the hospital for two days. Doesn't anyone care about him?" Her brisk questioning continues. "Do ya know why he's so sick? Look at him all black and blue. Can't you give him stronger medicine to get rid of that hurtin'?"

"I just increased his medication. It's a stronger amount and will make him comfortable tonight." I decide that now is the time to give Betsy more information. I sit back down on what has become my chair. I make eye contact with her and explain about Carter's blood infection. I don't mention the possibility of AIDS or cancer, nor do I hint at my efforts to assess his risk for AIDS. I swallow my uneasiness, what I suspect. "I hope to have more answers for you both in a couple of days," I say with as much resolve as I can summon.

"Call me as soon as ya know?" Betsy says and writes her phone numbers on a scrap of paper from her purse. Then she jumps up and grabs a plastic cup from the nightstand, holds the cup while Carter sips water through a straw.

The AIDS issue bounces around in my mind. I can't mention AIDS to Betsy until Carter is told. But what if he has AIDS, she needs to know so she can be tested. It is now five after four. There are three other patients to see. I stand up, wait for Carter to finish drinking. "Carter, tomorrow morning about nine o'clock I want to do a bone marrow biopsy in your pelvic bone to find out why your blood counts are low." I point to the biopsy site on my own pelvis and explain the procedure.

"Will I be awake?" Carter asks.

"Yes. But I'll give you lots of medicine to numb the bone." What if he has AIDS? There is always the chance of nicking my hand with the needle, although the probability is low. But there is always the fear. "I have lots of experience doing this type of biopsy." I realize I am reassuring myself.

"I guess I have to trust ya, Doc. Would ya let me stick needles in ya?" He laughs, then flinches. Betsy gives him a sip of her cola.

"Carter, I hate being stuck by needles," I say. "In medical school I fainted when I had blood taken from my arm. Now, whenever I have my blood tested, I lie down."

Both Betsy and Carter laugh. Then Betsy asks if she should be here for the biopsy.

"Betsy, go to work. We need the money. Doc and I won't need ya."

"Okay, tough guy." She chuckles and leans over to kiss Carter on his forehead. I wonder what her reaction will be if Carter has AIDS?

Carter asks her to bring him pajamas and some good food, points to her Wendy's cup.

"You feel like a burger and fries?"

"Maybe."

"I'll call ya after I leave school. Ya can give me your order then."

"Don't forget," he reminds her.

An overhead page gives me an excuse to leave. I say goodbye and go to the nurses' station. Betsy follows me. The noise level is dulled in the late afternoon, less chatter. We walk past patient transport carts and wheelchairs parked in the hallway.

"Doctor, how long will he live?" She whispers, a contrast with her earlier quick-fire questions.

"A long time maybe, depending on what's making him sick," I say, realizing this is probably not the truth.

"I can't believe this is happenin'. We just got married five months ago."

"How long have you known Carter?"

Betsy tells me that she's known him for two years. They met at a rodeo in Portsmouth. Her girlfriend's brother introduced them. They hit it off immediately. She was attracted to his humor, and they've always had lots of fun. He took a job selling auto parts in Chillicothe so they could be together.

"Even with the pain, he tries to lighten the mood," I say.

"That's Carter. Always kiddin' around." Tears well up in her eyes.

My pager beeps again. Knowing Betsy needs my attention I ignore the message.

"Does he have cancer?" she asks.

"I'm not sure. I should know in two days. Right now I want to focus on relieving his pain."

Carter's nurse walks up to Betsy and introduces herself. She extends her arm around Betsy's shoulder and walks her back toward Carter's room. I am relieved and use this moment to gather my thoughts before I see the next patient. This day has consumed me. I keep one eye on the clock but try to give patients my time. Who am I kidding? Why am I trying to give Betsy hope? Carter looks battered, smells. He is dying.

The next day I perform the bone marrow biopsy without problems and don't engage in much additional conversation. Two days later, I muster the courage to enter Carter's room in the late morning. I sit on the chair next to his bed. "Are you more comfortable?"

"Sometimes. The nurse said I was screamin' last night."

Get to the point I remind myself. "Carter, I have results from your tests."

"Bad?" he asks.

"You have some serious health problems."

He frowns at the pain of my words and closes his eyes.

I tell him that the bone marrow biopsy shows Hodgkin's disease, a type of cancer in his lymph nodes and bone marrow." He begins to cry. I rest my hand on his shoulder. I continue, "This type of cancer can be treated with chemotherapy. Sometimes the cancer disappears."

"Forever?"

"Sometimes." I take in a deep breath, prepare myself for the next part. "But there's another problem. You have AIDS." I remain quiet but am unsatisfied that I've told him this without a family member or close friend in the room to comfort him after I leave. Carter turns away from me. I notice how thin his black hair is on the back of his head. In this moment, it's not important how he got AIDS.

"Does Betsy know?" he asks.

"Not yet. Do you want to tell her or should I?"

"Ya tell her. God, I hope she's okay."

"She should be tested for AIDS."

A slight nod and more silence. There are no right words to fill these spaces.

The Brothers

ANN NEUSER LEDERER

I go to visit two brothers,
one eighty-eight, the other past ninety.
Scoured and shaved and smiling for the nurse.
Shoes shined, pants pressed and belted,
plaid shirts buttoned to the neck.

Past ninety takes his teeth out
when I ask to look in his mouth,
then he goes to bite me.
Both brothers chuckle.

This morning, says the young one,
he told his brother
while changing the diaper:
You're just like an old cow now.
I have to clean out your stall.
The brothers laughed and laughed.

The older brother adds:
My brother's a funny guy.
He don't say much,
but then
he comes out with something.

The Sisters
—Written in Love

ANTHONY FLEG

My watch said it was time to go,
But my heart spoke otherwise,
Fortunately, I listened to the latter
And went with Dr. Stuart to see
The Sisters

Miss Minnie and Miss Viola
Hailing from Georgia,
With ten scores of wisdom between them,
They spoke first, without words

Perfuming the room as we entered.
They began to tell of their aches and pains,
Joking about whether Dr. Stuart or I would be their "catch" for the day

When asked about the key to their longevity,
Viola answered, "God has been good to us,"
While their relative with them offered, "It is because they were good to their
  momma."

Which caused me to pause,
  Trying to shut off that medicalized, left-brain-oriented way of hearing
  that afflicts many of us in medicine,

They spoke not on the recipe for reaching the holy feat of triple digits,
But instead on the way to appreciate each day wholey,
  as something holy,
  They teach that the goal is not to reach an old age
  But instead is about how to be on your way there
    They remind us that the goal is not to avoid death
    But to fully embrace life

I am thankful,
I am refreshed,
Dr. Stuart and I leave smiling with our minds and hearts
If someone asks me why I am late
I'll simply say, "My teachers had something I needed to hear."

I Am the Handmaiden of the Lord

WILLIAM OREM

"Andeville Lake?" asked the young neurologist, crouched down with his palms held flat on his hips. Not that he needed the pose; this little girl was anything but threatened. Her own gaze went over the examination room in perceptive sweeps, stopping on the shiny cabinets, the wide-mouthed dispenser bottles, the poster with a dancing pachyderm. "I bet it's pretty up there, huh? Is it?"

The unspeaking girl had cherry-blonde hair that may not ever have been combed and tiny parts of her scalp showed through. Although she was almost a teenager, her forehead was pronounced like a child's, both it and her big plump cheeks scrubbed recently as if for a presentation. Underneath the dirt she had a pretty, boyish face and a frightening expression because late one evening Jesus had knocked on the screen of her window and asked if he could come inside. The neurologist stood up and went out of the room.

In the observation booth next door, a tall woman stood, her elbows resting tiredly on the glass. In the one-way light on the other side the girl sat swinging her legs.

"Andeville Lake is pretty far back," the neurologist said. "I know because I did some volunteer work in the Appalachians." He crossed his legs at the knee, a gesture intended to seem careless. "The roads are so bad we had to hike in. A lot of those places don't even have electricity."

"And is that related?" the woman asked. Her name was Candace Waller and she was a child psychologist. The neurologist understood her well. In four words she had just said to him: is this girl's cultural background of any clinical significance; if so, tell me how; if not, leave it. He offered a grin only partly conciliatory.

"Not specifically related. But she may have experienced malnourishment, or something, at some time."

"Does she show signs of malnourishment?"

"Not really."

"Well?" Her heavy glasses fixed on him carefully.

"For God's sake, Candy. She comes from the hills of West Virginia. You're the kid psychologist. That's all I wanted to say."

"It's an incestuous situation? That's what you're suggesting. Without wanting to say it."

"It could be, is what I'm suggesting. Don't put me on the couch because I make certain assumptions."

"Who signed the admittance form?"

"An aunt. She seemed afraid to admit she had brought the girl in here."

There was a sterile wait.

"You know I don't use a couch, Jim."

"I don't have anything obvious here other than reported hallucinations," the neurologist continued, with effort. "There's nothing physically wrong with her. Her body is small for her age, she may have an iron deficiency. But it isn't a seizure disorder."

"Who said it was seizure?"

"The referring physician, who isn't their family doctor because they aren't on any kind of plan. Actually he's the third person who's seen her; the first two sent her back to the aunt. Apparently visions of the risen Christ aren't so unusual in some parts. But she's not Joan of Arc, right? She's an eleven-year-old girl. And Jesus kept coming to her at night and showing her his wounds, and the next thing she's standing up in the middle of Sunday services and passing along these cryptic messages." He mused. "This girl has ecstasies, Candy. The old kind."

The neurologist waited for a response. Her had never found Candace Waller an easy read; she was tough, one of the toughest they had, and in her way one of the best. A relentless worker, the achiever's achiever. There was something behind it, though, some part of her person she didn't let through. She was unmarried, and he had never known her to date.

"Anyway, the aunt finally took her to a local," he continued. "The local referred her to a hospital, the hospital referred her out of the state, if you follow me. And eventually we got her."

"What's her name?"

He looked at a sheet. "Dorothy Geisen. Dot."

"Okay. And what has she said about Jesus?"

"Full sensory accordance: he walks, he talks. She can taste blood when she sees him. Divine blood, you know? He reveals mysteries to her, plans for the well-being of the cosmos. You want more?"

"No," Candace said, after a long pause. "I'm ready."

Within a minute or two she found, as usual, that she could successfully ignore the big silver eye of the one-way mirror and start to project an air of, if not quite normalcy, at least calm in front of the patient. When she was with a child she always thought of herself as Candy; not Dr. Waller, not Mom, not even Your Friend, because all those things were loaded with secret implications of which she could know nothing. Candy pulled up a swivel chair and, when Dot did not acknowledge her, followed the girl's stare.

"Do you like the silver?" she asked, taking hold of an aluminum tray. "That's pretty, isn't it?"

Dot smiled slowly, a little row of even teeth. None, for the record, missing.

"You're not a doctor," she said. "You're a woman."

"Well, that takes care of me. By the way, my name's Candace," she said, holding out one hand. "You can call me Candy if you like. Lots of people do."

"Candy."

"Yep. Like Candy Cane. What's your name?"

Dot looked away from the hand, uninterested.

"Dot, honey. Can I call you Dot? Is that okay? When I was a girl, just about your age, I had a imaginary friend named Polka Dot. I pretended she always wore a spotted dress. Anybody ever call you that?"

"I don't have friends."

"Sure you do. Some people you know from school maybe?"

Dot rolled her eyes in what Candace thought a remarkably adult gesture. She was about to speak again when the girl turned abruptly and began staring at her, staring so hard that for a moment Candace thought she was going to be shouted at. It had happened plenty of times. Then in a kind of revelation she realized it wasn't she herself that was being analyzed; Dot had taken an interest in her glasses. She took them off, passed them into the little hands. Unwashed hands, the fingernails bitten. Dot took them without comment, turning them in the light. Photophilia?

"They leave a line on my nose."

"Do you live in this city?" Dot asked irrelevantly.

"I do now. I grew up in New York. How about if you tell me about where you live?"

"Oh. Nowhere."

I'm nobody. Who are you? "I heard you live in Andeville. Isn't that right?"

Dot sighed ambiguously and looked back over at the window. Her feet picked up their abstracted rhythm.

Candace proceeded with the examination; if Dot wanted to speak, she would speak. Her work had given her enough experience with trying to pry secrets out of locked drawers to know that one didn't press beyond a point. She had crossed the point, once terribly, with a child who had been forced to have oral sex with her brother and who then equated being asked to speak with being told to open her mouth. That girl had gone into hysterics after too much prying, and Candace had left the room shaken deeply, feeling like she had just smacked the little streaming face.

Instead she looked closely at the girl now before her. There was a small tic above the left brow, random occurrences; the mouth hung a little slack. Maybe; but it was far from conspicuous. She had seen girls look this way from nothing more than insomnia.

"Can you touch my fingers if I move them like this? You try it. Take your hand out and try it, okay? I'll move them like this and you reach out and touch them. I'll bet somebody downstairs already asked you to do this. That's too easy."

After ten minutes or so Candace pretty much knew there was nothing glaringly wrong with this backwoods Virginian girl to which she could point. As predicted, Dot was largely uncommunicative, doing what she was asked but unwilling to comment further; but she did not show any markings of the oftentimes obvious physical side of psychosis. And the only way to find what was broken, Candace thought in one of her mother's home truisms, was to touch where it hurt.

With terrific slowness she began combing out Dot's hair with her fingers: entirely a contact gesture, as the hair was grown at several spots into inseparable cables. The girl did not resist, and Candace continued offhandedly talking about her own childhood in Brooklyn. She told about how in the summertime the fire department opened the hydrants for one day and made a stream that ran through the middle of the neighborhood, and the sunlight shone on that stream and she would sit on a fire escape and watch the children next door playing in it. She told about how she taught herself to raise geraniums in a pot on her windowsill, only you had to be careful because the birds would come by and pick at the flowers when they came out. She went on about her high school in Brooklyn that was run by the Sisters of Jesus, and then it occurred to her with complete unexpectedness that in all the stories she told of herself as a girl she was always alone.

"I see him in the nighttime," Dot said frankly.

"Oh?" Candace said, surprised by her own thoughts and trying to keep her tone as neutral as possible. For a moment the girl in front of her almost sounded as if she were bragging.

"Yes. Jesus the Lord and Master comes in my window and he comes by my bed and he stands there and he tells me things, yes, and he shows me things too."

"Does he? Well, and what happens then?"

"He tells me to put my fingers in his sides and in the holes in his palms, yes, and to believe. He says he only wants me to love him."

"Is that nice?"

"And he shows me where his bloody holes are and where they tear his clothes. And they laugh at him, to mock and to deride. And they take him to Golgotha, which is, the place of the skull. And he dies and takes me with him to Gehenna, which is, the place of burning. Of harrowing."

Dot's eyes had become liquid ash, running wild; the transformation was unbelievably swift. She turned and looked at Candace with sudden and startling lucidity, as if she had cognitively grown five years in as many seconds.

"Oh? And is he a nice man or a mean man?" Candace tried. She could hear her own heart rate increasing, fought to keep it out of her face. "What do you think?"

"And he shows me the end, which is written upon a great scroll that is at once the sky and the sea. And the moon is like unto my blood. And the sky is the color of the earth, that is judgment. For the Holy of Holies has been defiled. Yes, and the ram with one thousand seeing eyes opens there the seal that is the fourth and the sacred of the Lord is shown . . ."

"Dot?" Candace asked. "Honey?"

"And they depart from me you swineherds and you unbefaithful, *ye that knew me not, when I was naked, and afraid, into that terrible place which is prepared by Satan and all his angels. . . .*"

The old man in the waiting room had an awkward condition of the spine, which made him stand in such a position as one might if considering a golf putt before actually bending to the task. His skull was proud and granular looking with a thin stubble of hair that swung around it like a monk's, and his clothes were of a consistent vague color. He was Dorothy Geisen's father.

"Monkey brains," he hissed, sneering through soft lips. His eyes bristled with hatred for the examining physician and Candace Waller as they had for the attendant nurses he had found on the way in and the lab chief, a stout, proud man named Attin, to whom they had taken him. His perpetual stoop made the animosity seem wicked, like a physical threat. But his obvious physical weakness turned the threat tragic, furiously absurd. Behind him stood the frightened aunt, her face and her clothes dark and rumpled looking, her spirit withered and gone. She stared at her handbag in misery.

"You people are trying to put monkey brains in my daughter," the man growled. "I know! I know!" The fingers on one hand flexed in and out at his side where the arm hung straight, and if they had reached significantly out of his coat sleeve he might have been thought to be making a fist. "You can't keep her here. She's coming back with me. I want you to give her to me now. Now."

"Mr. Geisen, this is Dr. Parkes," the lab chief began, gesturing to the neurologist.

"I don't care who the hell he is! I don't care a stitch for any one of you! You tell me where my daughter is now and you give her back to me! She won't get any monkey brains . . ."

"Mr. Geisen," Candace fired sharply, coming in close. "I've just been talking to your daughter. You should understand—"

The old man spat in her face.

"Bitch!" he shouted. "You bitch! You keep your filthy hands off my girl. You—"

"All right, Dr. Waller, Dr. Parkes, I'm asking you to step into another room," the lab chief said loudly, taking them by the arms. "I'm asking this now. Come on."

As soon as they had moved away, the old man quieted down but lost none of his bundled rage, still stepping back and forth on the rug like a fighter between rounds. The neurologist put a hand on Candace's arm and she took it off.

"I'm quite all right," she said, wiping her face.

"The problem is, he has custody," the neurologist said in an excited whisper, as if somehow guilty of his information. "That old Jethro. He just came crashing in, demanding her, and nobody can fight it. We know there's nothing wrong with the girl. And the aunt has no legal rights over her, because it turns out she's not even a real part of the family. There's no way the Chief is going to hold on to this."

"Nothing wrong?" Candace said, incredulous. "Did you just say there's nothing wrong with her?"

"Grossly wrong. Physically wrong. You know what I mean."

"Did you listen to that girl, Jim? Did you hear what she was saying to me just now? Did you?"

"Let me ask you one," the neurologist said. "Do you think old man Geisen here is Jesus by night? This guy who can't even . . . I mean look at him."

"I think that girl is troubled. Very troubled. You yourself said malnourishment."

"And you said no."

"Well, what the hell is he doing going off and leaving her with a friend anyway? I think we can claim neglect."

"No, now *you* listen to the question," the neurologist said. "Could you say to a legal counsel that this girl shows undisputable signs of being abused by that man? Do you think he's feeding her drugs?"

She gritted her teeth.

"No. I don't think those things right now. But I only just met the patient, Doctor."

"Then what can we say? She's not 'the patient' just because we think she should be. Somebody would call it a religious dispute. Say we're administering Prozac to shut out the voice of God."

"She needs us," Candace faltered, her voice suddenly quiet.

"I'm sorry?"

"You don't know what it . . . what being a girl is like. You don't know. When you're alone, at that age . . . and you would do anything . . ."

"I'm not hearing this."

"She has a blessing!" the old man shouted from the next room. He was cupping his dry hands together around his croaking voice, making himself heard like a wilderness prophet. "She has a blessing!"

They missed the four o'clock bus, and the black woman behind the glass booth suggested that "if you in *such* a hurry" they could take a series of three city buses that would get them roughly to the same place where there would be another train leaving close to the time the third bus would arrive there. She smiled down at the little girl, the wavy glass distorting her mouth.

After three blocks they found the bus stop and they took the bus, sitting on the front seat which resembled red vinyl and was torn. Someone had written on it with a blue pen: *Stella M.* The unfinished phrase bothered the old man and he sat, his back cramping down into the awkward seat and his knotty hands on the rail, gritting angrily at the nonsense words. They could have been the speaking voice of the city, where evil and senselessness were fused.

The second bus was late in coming and then an electronic church bell with a loudspeaker was ringing the hour of four and it hadn't come at all, so he took the girl, who had been fingering a ball of tin foil in a flower pot, and they began walking down the hot sidewalk. His fingers were calloused and weak and she had to hold onto him with the tighter grip. With his other hand he reached into his jacket pocket and at the tips of his nails ran along the edge of a small ticket, a return, the remaining half of the one he had bought coming into Union Station. There was also the remains of a small note written by that woman they called the girl's aunt for convenience sake, which explained her actions with a few words underlined and had been left on the small coffee table in the kitchen under a sugar spoon. He had torn it in his anger and then taped it back together for no good reason. Now he removed it from his pocket and dropped it onto the walk, letting it skitter away in a gust of foul air.

"Those people in there," the old man said, as if talking to the passing cracks on the sidewalk or perhaps to the young black men, wearing strange, loose clothing, seated on a curb and watching the old man and his daughter go by. "Did you tell them about what happens at nighttime? What happens with you?"

The girl bobbed her head nonspecifically. She was watching the cars as they nosed each other's ends like a clumsy herd.

"Because they would not understand a thing like that. They may put you in those devil machines, but they never would understand a thing like that. And there's no sense in you telling what someone won't understand." He shook her wrist. "The Bible says *he that hath ears, let him hear.* Do you understand?"

They walked on. The sun was glowering over the rich and ruinous buildings, an angry assertion. After a while he spoke again.

"Those machines they put you in," he said. "They didn't touch you or nothing? In the machines?"

The girl shook her head around, her hair dangling.

"Before God," the old man said. During the trip up he had been so enraged and so afraid for his daughter that the feelings moved inside him like a physical pain. They walked and his legs were tired and the hurting at the joints; he had been walking and riding and walking again in this senseless collection of street debris since early that morning and he hurt now, all over, a deep hurt at the bone. His pace was slowing but the girl didn't seem to notice, moving and tugging at his holding hand like a balloon on the end of a string.

"Candy," she said. "Candy, candy, candy, candy, candy, candy."

"All right, all right," the old man said, wanting her to see him angered but secretly pleased just to hear her voice. "If you are good."

Cattleman

MICHAEL R. ROSMANN

Kent raised the manure-splattered tailgate of the livestock trailer to let his cows enter the chute into the Farmers Livestock Auction stockyards. This was the last truckload of his 130 cows that were scheduled to be sold at today's auction. Most of the red and white cows hurriedly tramped down the sloped chute to reach the more solid footing of the concrete alleyway leading to their pens. There they would wait for prospective buyers to inspect them. Kent was familiar with each animal as she passed and knew all their ear tag numbers and names.

He remembered how he helped Sally give birth to twins in April 2003. Sally's first calf was coming with one front leg turned backward. Despite Sally's contractions, Kent pushed the calf's head and chest back into her uterus and reached inside to pull up the errant leg. After grasping both front feet, he quickly pulled the wet calf into the outside world. The second calf was less fortunate, for Kent discovered that its umbilical cord had become twisted earlier during its detained emergence.

Wincing from the hollow feeling in his stomach, Kent watched as Belle scrambled down the chute, and he remembered that she had produced the high-selling bull in his annual production sale twice in the past five years. "I'll miss you." Then Molly came to the trailer doorway and briefly locked onto his gaze as she gingerly placed one hoof ahead of the other into the chute. They had an eleven-year relationship. "Sorry, old girl."

When all the cattle were unloaded and chased into their holding pens by the sale hands, Kent visited the auction office to tell the clerks that he had delivered all his cows. With a Styrofoam cup of steaming coffee quivering in his thick hand, Kent headed to the holding pens in the adjoining shed to take a last look at his pets.

Several farmers were exchanging comments while leaning on the corral gates and scraping their boots on the gate planks in front of his cows. Two laughing boys swatted at each other with their caps and a few girls—less rambunctious—meandered up and down the alleys while their dads checked out the cattle and shared a few words with people they knew. Kent talked to several potential buyers, as he remembered folks who had purchased bulls or heifers previously. Most complimented Kent about how his stock had improved their herds. Several uttered comments about not being able to afford any additions this fall. They commiserated about the awful beef prices and hoped that many buyers would show up at today's auction.

Kent's red-bodied white-faced cattle were the major feature of the sale, which included 2,600 cattle of all sizes, ages, weights, and colors. Kent wondered for a moment if he'd made the right choice when he opted to specialize in Hereford cattle twenty-three years earlier. He and his father had tried a number of breeds. They found that the gentle, thrifty, accommodating Herefords worked best in the rolling hills of grass and timber of western Iowa.

"I remember your top pen-of-five heifers at the Tri-State Beef Futurity," a fellow Hereford breeder from a neighboring county proffered while clearing his throat. "When was that?"

"In '98 and again in '99," Kent said; those were years he'd remember on his deathbed.

"Should bring you some buyers?"

"Maybe," Kent said, again aware of the queasiness in his gut.

Retreating into self-absorption, Kent recalled with disgust that many city folks were turning away from red meat. He wondered how Maureen was feeling; she was probably already waiting for him to join her in the arena bleachers. She was as worried as he about having had to cash in their retirement account to cover debts. Next year they would both reach sixty years. He recalled last evening's conversation with Todd Holstrup of the Conservative Savings Bank. Todd wished him well but said the bank needed all the income from the sale of the cattle to reduce the unpaid loan from 2004. Kent considered himself another year older and another year deeper in debt.

The loudspeaker in the sale barn implored potential buyers to assemble in the arena surrounding the sale ring. Kent took a final stroll down the alleyway in front of the wooden gates corralling his cows. At the last pen Molly stuck her nose through the planks of the fence. Kent patted her on the head and recalled the previous February when Molly gave birth unexpectedly early. Sometimes older cows unintentionally abort their calves prematurely during particularly harsh weather conditions to muster strength in their own bodies. This had happened to Molly. She hadn't joined the herd as he unrolled the big round bales of hay on hoof-packed snow with his old Farmall 460 tractor. Scouring the landscape, he spotted her almost a half mile away, close to the timber. A terribly cold day, the northerly winds blew thirty miles per hour creating a forty degrees below zero wind chill. Kent drove his tractor to see what was happening with Molly. Just as he suspected, she was standing next to the frozen body of a slightly premature calf. He didn't bother to check the fetus's gender. In response to his calls, Molly trudged behind the Farmall until they reached the shelter of the comfortable old calving barn.

The next day Kent presented Molly with a black-and-white-spotted calf that he purchased from a dairy farmer who routinely sold baby bull calves at the sale barn. When Kent plopped the calf onto the wheat straw in Molly's pen, she looked at him as if to say, "Why are you doing this and what do you expect me to do?" Molly politely blocked the hungry newcomer from her swollen udder, slowly shoving her rear legs back and forth. Kent approached Molly's head and scratched her behind her poll. He looked her in the eye and pronounced, "I'm sorry you lost your calf. This is the best I can do. Won't you take care of him?" Molly gazed at Kent and then at the new prospect, considering her options. After a few seconds, she firmly planted both hind feet on the ground and allowed the spotted calf to nurse. Tears welled in Kent's eyes; there was mutual respect and trust. They had taken care of each other in different ways for many years.

The sale announcer was urging all bidders to register for the auction and to find seats in the sale arena. Kent rejoined the crowd, realizing that he needed to be available to answer questions in case the auctioneer wanted to know about his cattle's pedigrees and backgrounds. As he plodded toward the sale ring, Molly mooed softly. With each distancing step, Molly bellowed more affirmatively.

A heavyset neighboring farmer in coveralls lumbered to catch up with Kent and protested, "Kent, why is that cow bellerin'?"

Kent stopped in his tracks, turned, and responded, "She's wondering what she did wrong that she should have to be sold."

The hefty man momentarily paused and put a hand on Kent's shoulder. "Yeah, it's too bad," he murmured.

Shivering, Kent struggled to maintain his composure. He remembered the words of his psychologist whom he had consulted last week for his depression. "Why don't you keep a few cows for yourself; they'll help you maintain your self-respect."

Kent recalled how hard he and his father had worked to set fences around their 310 acres of brome grass and to segregate the pasture from their row crops. He contemplated how he and Maureen had put three children through college and had taken care of Kent's father who was no longer able to help with the chores because of his stroke. The drought of 2003 and high winds caused greensnap to cut his corn yield to half the normal production. That fall the bottom fell out of the cattle market as many drought-stricken cow-calf operations flooded the market with cows and calves. Kent regretted not having sold some of his brood cows when low cattle prices continued into 2004 and 2005. He recalled, too, how frightened he was by the prospect of having to pay both the loan principal and interest when he didn't have the cash on hand. Federal crop insurance payments on the deficient corn production helped a little, but there was no insurance program for his livestock needs, only more USDA loans. They made the wisest decisions they could at the time, and Maureen seldom questioned him. They thought that they could ride out this low cattle price cycle. Kent considered his banker's frequent worried telephone calls and summons to the bank office.

The stout neighbor loosened his grip on Kent's shoulder. The men parted and Kent headed toward the sale ring. After a few steps, he halted. Slowly, deliberately, he took a ballpoint pen from his left shirt pocket and wrote down several numbers on a slip of paper. At the door of the sale ring, he handed the paper to the ring man and said, "Hold these cows and put them in a pen in the back of the barn."

The ring manager hesitated, then nodded and ordered the waiting sale hands to carry out his orders.

Kent climbed to where Maureen had saved him a spot in the wooden bleachers. She slipped her left hand over Kent's right fist as his cows entered the sale ring. The auctioneer chanted his calls. Maureen's warm hand squeezed Kent's curled fingers every time the gavel rang down on the podium and the auctioneer announced, "Sold!" A few minutes and it was all over.

Kent was sweating and Maureen was still clasping his right hand firmly as they descended and then weaved through the onlookers standing in the aisle next to the exit sign. As soon as they reached the rutted parking lot, Kent began to tremble. Sobs gushed forth. Questions tumbled in his head. "What did I do wrong? Will Todd be mad because I didn't sell all my cows?" Next week was his equipment sale. Could he go on? The arthritis in his hands and the torn rotator cuff in his left shoulder were small pains in comparison to having to sell his cattle and farming equipment. Would he be able to preserve the homestead that was so heavily mortgaged? Maureen took his head and held it to her shoulder.

Two hours later, Kent and Maureen drove the half-filled semitruck down the lane toward home. Kent backed the trailer to the unloading dock next to the calving barn. Sally was the first to step out of the trailer. Belle followed. Molly, slower than the rest, was last. As she thrust her head through the rear trailer opening, she stared at Kent. Their eyes met. Then Molly tossed her head and mooed as she took a step. Kent shuddered, then grinned, as he understood Molly's gentle rebuke.

Call

MICHAEL PERRY

We nearly made the millennium without 911. Until 1999, whether for a grass fire or a heart attack, you dialed a seven-digit number that rang in the homes of everyone on the department. A "phone bar," it was called. Now we're summoned by pager, but some tradition survives: The old-timers still call the old number, and the first person to the fire hall still triggers the water-tower siren. We all come running. Someone is calling for help. It's that simple, really, and that profound.

On a frozen December night, the pager goes off when I am on the edge of my bed, having just killed the light. A woman stopped to visit her grandfather and found him flat on the bedroom floor. In the parlance of the dispatcher, he is un-responsive. In the parlance of mechanics, his heart has stalled. Mine, however, is now pumping blood enough for two men. Light switch, pants, shirt, boots, I'm on my way. Grab a jacket on the porch, and thump down the backyard footpath.

On a dead run, it takes me roughly thirty seconds to get from my house to the fire hall. A little longer if have to punch through frozen crust and hurdle the snowbank at the Legion Hall. Once, on a warm summer night, I cut across the neighboring lot on the dead run at 2 A.M., tripped, and was airborne be-fore I remembered the concrete foundation of the abandoned filling station. I experienced one of those extruded moments produced when startle precedes impact—when your car is skidding toward another car, for instance, or when a flowerpot is headed for the tiles—and time hypertrophies. Nanoseconds become roomy and habitable. The forces of physics continue apace, but our synapses fire with such stroboscopic precision that afterward we can't believe we thought all we thought. I recall gliding in the pitch-dark night, recognizing what had just happened, considering the history of the long-gone building, the smell of the grass, the pleasant feeling of suspension and motion, the push of the air on my face, the arc of descent, the palpable bulk of the giant sugar maple I knew stood to my left. I visualized my hand, cocked at the wrist, reaching out for the ground. I entertained a series of omniscient stop-motion views revealing the orientation of my body in space. In free fall, I calculated the likely angle of impact and prepared to roll with it. I thought of my father, telling me that a bullet shot from a perfectly level gun would hit the ground at the same time as a bullet simply dropped from the same height as the barrel. It's a mind-twister, accepting that horizontal motion doesn't extend hang time. And then I hit, tucked, rolled, and was just as quickly on my feet, running again, remembering to duck the neighbor's clothesline.

That old foundation is gone now, replaced by a yellow prefab, and so tonight I run straight out my backyard, through eight inches of snow. The temperature stands at dead zero. I feel as if I'm pushing my face through rubbing alcohol. My cheeks stiffen, have the feel of butter hardening. With every inhalation, the hair in my nostrils freezes. The village is still, the stillness intensified by the cold. Christmas is a few weeks away. Here and there the neighborhood glows with illuminated plastic snowmen, electrified garlands, and strings of icicle lights. At the house across the street, a four-foot glowing Santa slumps against the door in a nimbus of red. From here he looks drunk.

I clear the snowbank at a good clip, cross Elm Street, and punch the combination into the fire door. In the summer, it's *click, click, click,* and you're in. Tonight the works are seized with cold. It feels as if I am pushing the buttons through taffy. I expect to see Pam or Jack or the Beagle, but no one is around. I'm pretty sure the address is just west of town, but the rule is, you don't go anywhere before you find it on the map, so I run to the meeting room and check the wall to be sure. Yep. There it is. I spin on my heel, flick the garage door opener, start the van, and, hoping someone else is going to show up, let it idle while I pull on a pair of rubber gloves. Nobody shows. I'm going solo. I hit the lights and hit the road.

The calls blindside you, always. You will prepare and prepare, and you will never be prepared. We are never ready, and our patients are never ready. Over the years, I have developed a visceral reaction to families and victims expressing surprise at tragedy. Why are we surprised? Why do we forget we are mortal? Bad, bad things happen everywhere, every day. Humans, for better or worse, harbor this feeling that we—individually—are special. A patch of ice or a pea-sized blood clot makes a mockery of that illusion in a heartbeat. We are not special at all. I hear people on scene saying, "Why? Why?" and the answer is, there is no why. Ambulance work will exacerbate your inner existentialist.

My brother John made a call, he came busting in the kitchen, and the first thing that hit him was a palpable wave of cigarette smoke and bacon grease. A man was spilled backward on the floor, his chair upended. His plate was mounded with half-finished eggs and sausage links. His cigarettes had slipped from his shirt pocket. His white belly protruded like risen dough. And his wife looked at my brother, and she said, "I don't understand . . . he's never been sick a day in his life."

And John says he remembers his first thought was, Well, he's sick now.

Alone in the van, I have a ball in my gut. I can already feel the eyes that will turn to me as I step through the door. The eyes will be stricken and hopeful, and I will throw myself into doing what I've been trained to do, not so much out of hope as a means of avoiding those eyes, because I know the man who lives here, and I know his health is poor, and I have a terribly accurate idea of the likelihood of my doing him any good. I step through the patio doors and one woman is tearful in the kitchen, pointing down to the end of the trailer, and in the bedroom, the man is flat on the floor and another woman is doing CPR, and as soon as I enter the bedroom she stands, backs away from the man, and bursts into tears. The bed has been pushed aside. A half-eaten muffin rests on the windowsill.

I strip my stethoscope out of the pack now and listen for a heartbeat. In the midst of the mess and panic, you plug the earpieces in, press the bell against the still chest, and listen. You are hoping to hear audible hydraulics from a fist's worth of muscle. You are scanning for life's backbeat. The lup-dup groove. A little heavier on the dup. That most ineffable iamb.

Nothing. I place an oral airway. It is a simple plastic device that keeps the tongue from the back of the throat, allows air to pass through the mouth. I resume CPR. Headlights sweep the window, and shortly my mother is kneeling beside me. She has a defibrillator and a Combitube. We attach the defib pads and fire up the machine. The line that should be bouncing across the screen is flat, flat, flat. Doing chest compressions with one hand, I grab my radio from the floor and call Chetek 245, to give them an update. When they answer, I can hear their siren in the background.

"This is two-forty-five, go ahead, New Auburn first responders." I recognize the voice as Karen, an EMT I've taken shifts with for years.

"Two-forty-five, be advised we have an elderly adult male patient who suffered an unwitnessed cardiac arrest. . . . CPR was in progress . . . at this time the patient is . . . is . . ." And then I lock up. For some reason, when I try to come up with the term we use in these situations—PNB, for "pulseless nonbreather"—I draw a complete blank. The only term I can summon is "Nebraska sign," the old EMS chestnut equating the patient's EKG tracing to the topography of the Cornhusker state. Not the sort of line you want to use over the airwaves or in front of family. I blurt out the next thing that comes to mind.

"Ahh . . . this patient is a *flat-liner.*"

After a little pause, Karen 10-4s me. There is a grin in her voice. It seems inappropriate, and unlike her. Later, she says when they heard that "flat-liner" business, they got the giggles in spite of the situation, because they wanted to know exactly what TV show was it I thought I was on?

This selection is from Michael's best-selling memoir *Population 485: Meeting Your Neighbors One Siren at a Time* (Harper Collins, 2002).

Learning to Walk the Healer's Path

ERIK BRODT

Three minutes and thirty seconds remained in the fourth quarter of the Minnesota Section 6A boys' basketball final. Showcasing a fake plant step, our All-State point guard sends his opponent to the floor again. Dribbling around the flopping contender, number 5 pulls up and sinks a fifteen-foot jumper to put Cass-Lake up by four. But there is a turn of fate. Floating down from his jump shot, our point guard landed on the foot of another player, twisting his ankle inward and sending him to the floor in agony. Hearts dropped with the crowd's deep gasp. Silence. I gulped nervously as my time was at hand. I composed myself and strolled onto the court to help our star as thousands looked on.

"Three minutes and thirty seconds!" she shouted as I threw myself into my disaster gown. "Estimated time of arrival, three minutes and thirty seconds!" My hands quivered cold with sweat as my fingerprints formed though my latex gloves. Confusion rested on my shoulder. I didn't know what, but I could feel something horrible happening.

That day, now eternally etched into my mind, had begun as a splendid day. Each step was light, walking between medicine clinic and the women's health ward to visit a laboring mother and evaluate a baby I had delivered in the morning. Wearing a wide grin of connection and accomplishment, I fought to contain the giddy chuckles of becoming a doctor. When all is well, being a doctor is bliss. Pulling the hospital door, it didn't budge. Puzzling. Why was our rural hospital locked in the middle of the day? My pager sounded, I was needed in the ER immediately. March 21 will never be another day to me. No day will.

As a third-year medical student I performed a nine-month rural clerkship at North Country Regional Hospital in Bemidji, Minnesota. I chose Bemidji to be close to my family and the three largest Minnesota Chippewa Reservations. I am Anishinaabe (Chippewa) and it was the perfect opportunity for me to invest in the Native community during medical school. Little did I know how profound an impact the experience would have on me, especially on the afternoon when a young man entered Red Lake High School, shooting thirteen people and killing eight, including himself.

Two days earlier, I had looked proudly on the young men of the Cass Lake-Bena basketball team as they were welcomed home to the reservation following a successful state tournament. In the ER I found myself staring at young, Native men, all victims of the tragedy in Red Lake. My mind raced and my stomach curdled sour. Do I know this kid? Oh, no. Does he remember me? There is ——. I hope her child is all right. Which one of hers is behind the curtain? Recounting what I saw would not serve anyone justice; just know that I now understand the meanings of "gruesome" and "horror." I was devastated. I played basketball with their brothers, knew their faces from powwows, and remembered their passions and joys from sports events. When you are related—no matter how distant—when you are community, no matter how close or wide, when you know the life and family that goes with the mangled face, you stop. Everything stops.

I grew up rural, but I never realized the challenges of providing care to a close-knit community until I lived it from a provider perspective. Initially I was shocked by the shooting, then the media frenzy. However, once the last patient was discharged and the camera lights dimmed, the community remained—remained with many questions and in need of healing. So did I. My life floated without direction or breeze. I hovered in suspended animation, cold and alone.

My stomach simmered the awful sights, smells, and sounds of that day. My thoughts and dreams replayed the contrasting images and emotions of victory and violence: young men full of life and hope and young men lying dead and still. I was sick, hollow veined, confused by the instant flashes of beauty and horror. One day we were living the rural Hoosier's dream; I woke the next day in a nightmare. The pendulum swung swiftly. Our community climate was a schizophrenic storm of emotions. The joys of athletic victory and Reservation pride were short lived and the heartache of tragedy held stationary. A soft, gray rain fell for months.

The physicians faced challenges in waves. Initially stabilization and emergent skills were needed, followed by communication and counseling sessions with families. As the weeks turned and the months passed, the most difficult challenges arose: addressing the many faces of grief in one's self and the community.

I watched as many banded together and found comfort in numbers. Others withdrew and searched within. Some found solace in addictions. During my last four months I could not help but wonder if the events of March 21 were connected to each new case of anxiety or depression. Or if pending divorce, job loss, car accident, or belly pain were the end result of some hope lost after the shooting. I felt some hope lost, perhaps soul loss. Rural physicians, like their patients, spare anonymity and feel much of the impact of community events—jubilant or tragic. The question for me turned into one of reconciliation.

How am I to flourish in medicine as a young practitioner when I find myself so disconnected and disenchanted by human violence? How am I going to heal? This time AND the next time? As a Native physician, how am I going to approach dark events within the Native community? Medicine quickly teaches a young doctor there is plenty of joy and heartache. Will I be able to withstand repeated heartache striking close to home? How can I continue my course for positive social change?

Too many funerals happened that spring—Christian and traditional Native. The community turned to spiritual leaders, counselors, and physicians for healing. As for me, I left town. The weight of the shooting was crushing me and I could not stay any longer to keep reliving the events. All the constant reminders of the shooting—the media, the hospital, and town—quickly faded from my rearview mirror as I drove toward melting snow and robins. Hours later I arrived at an Ojibwe language and culture retreat. An elder friend of mine was there for similar reasons. We both needed reprieve. By sharing our hurts and joys with one another, a bond formed between two healers. Away from the steaming edge of a boiling ocean, I was able to start processing my experience with another who understood my pain. We talked for minutes, which became hours. The hours morphed into car rides north of Bemidji where we would sit, listen, laugh, and begin to heal. Finally, the burdens in my chest began to lift.

Later that year I sought guidance from another friend—a man who heals people in traditional Ojibwe ways. We sat around a healing fire waiting on the rocks to glow brilliant orange. Staring into the woods, he began to share his experiences as a healer and how he approaches the dark events in the lives of those he helps. The forest hushed while he shared his ways of staying on a good path when darkness hits too close. My breaths became conscious and intentional. He enforced the necessity of healing the healer. Each syllable chimed with each blazing clink of the firing rocks, "You need to develop thick skin."

I shuddered. At first I did not understand, thinking he was encouraging me to become callous and disconnected from the community. This was the opposite of my life vision in medicine. As I listened to his words, I realized the "thick skin" was more like a protective glove. Not a hard, impenetrable shell, but a tight barrier wrapping around and flowing with my humanity. The thin layer would continue to permit me to feel—feel warmth and touch—but provide a cushion from inflictions when asked to care for people in dark extremes. He guided me to seek out necessary experiences and skills to flame-forge my own gloves, to be equipped to meet the dynamic challenges to care for a Native community. I have taken the challenge like a moth to a flame.

Many things have since changed; children are growing up and dear elders have passed. I am weeks and months further from March 2005, but the lessons learned are as crisp as September skies. The joys and heartaches I experience each day as a young doctor are being cast into a layer around me, thus permitting me to heal myself and others. With advice to seek balance and develop "thick skin," I have become more humane with my patients, and them with me. Wearing my experience-woven skin over my healing hands gives me the strength to endure and the confidence to succeed in providing essential care when life turns cold or springs bliss.

Asking the Right Questions

THERESE ZINK

"Two blocks into my paper route and I can't peddle my bike," Joe complains. He tells us the pain started when he was playing Hacky Sack. He rotates his hip out and balances on his left foot, his right knee protrudes from his denim shorts like a doorknob. Ankle-high red tennis shoes squeak on the linoleum floor. I marvel at his flexibility considering all the pain he describes. "Sometimes my knee locks up and I have to massage it to release it," Joe says and demonstrates. "Twenty Ibuprofen in two hours doesn't touch it!" His blonde ponytail flips from one shoulder to the other.

Joe and Doug, the patient and the medical student, are in their early twenties. Both are tall; their clothes hang on them like a dress shirt drapes a hanger. Doug listens intently, making notes on his clipboard from his post on the exam room stool. Near the end of a nine-month rural rotation during his third year of medical school, he has seen patients at the local hospital, clinic, and nursing home and learned about the community's health issues. He's rented a trailer home in the town's trailer park. As faculty in the Rural Physician Associate Program at the medical school, I am here for one of six visits to assess his progress, observing his interactions with patients and doctors, the professor monitoring the student.

Doug methodically uncovers the how, when, why, where, and what about Joe's pain, what makes it better and what makes it worse. Shifting his focus between his notes and Joe, he pauses and runs his long fingers through his short brown hair. I hold my tongue during the pregnant silences and Doug always comes through with the appropriate next question. I quietly applaud him.

Joe claims to smoke a pack a day in the summer and increases to almost a carton a day in the winter. However, neither his clothes nor his body reek of cigarette smoke. There are no tobacco stains on his fingers. Quitting? He's thought about it, but it's not a priority right now.

Alcohol consumption? Two drinks a week; goes through a bottle of Jack Daniels in about six months. No pot now, because his girlfriend told him to stop. No other drugs or pills.

Joe's life adventures are entertaining: snowboarding shenanigans in the winter; having a friend tow him on his skateboard behind a car; asking a friend to run into his van at thirty miles per hour, "for the kick." He seems to relish our attention and Doug's direct, and easy manner puts Joe at ease.

Joe readjusts his ball cap, rotating it on his head when he talks about his girlfriend. He likes her "a lot." "We've had sex for a few months." Shyly he admits to no protection.

So far, Doug has documented Joe's history of present illness, past medical history, and family history and is working through social history. As Doug concludes the interview and prepares to conduct the physical exam, I decide to interrupt and ask Joe where he lives.

"In my van," he responds.

At this, Doug's gaze locks with mine and he settles back on his stool, crosses his legs and begins a new line of questioning, probing where Joe gets money for food and cigarettes. Again, I am proud of Doug, having observed his maturation from student to physician during the nine months.

Joe tells us that his sixteen-year old girlfriend is pregnant. "She wants to have my baby," he says, shrugging his bony shoulders and staring at his tennis shoes. "She's my first girlfriend in two years. I'm in love."

The sticky strands of a complex psychosocial situation envelop Doug and me. Joe willingly answers more of Doug's questions.

He drank a lot, until his New Year's "revolution." His father "whooped" him for years with a belt and other convenient home implements. Recently he threatened him with a two by four and then Joe moved into his van. "We're not talking now." Joe runs an informal taxi service around town. "Business has been great with the high price of gas." He tells us that he can't get a job anywhere. "Even Wal-Mart! I just can't do the work." He mumbles something about Social Security disability.

The real reason for his visit is now apparent to me, but Doug's expression doesn't change. I wonder if he's picked up on this. Joe climbs up onto the exam table and Doug performs a thorough lower extremity exam. He describes his findings—everything normal—and tells Joe that he's going to talk with the physician and will be back soon. "Any other questions?" Doug asks before moving toward the door.

Joe shrugs.

Dr. Jones, Doug's preceptor, is in his early forties. He looks up from his computer as we walk into the room. The papers and journals on his desk are organized in neat piles. "You know how many patients I saw while you were in there?" he laughs.

"We just saved you a lot of time," I say.

Despite his busy schedule, Dr. Jones integrates teaching. He has encouraged Doug's independence, allows him to take a stab at a patient's assessment and plan, and gently corrects him if he is off target. "So what you got?" Dr. Jones says with a grin.

Doug clears his throat and presents the case: "This is a thrill-seeking twenty-year-old who smokes, drinks, has a pregnant girlfriend, takes physical risks, and had an abusive childhood that continues. He's here for knee pain, but the exam is normal, and I think his real agenda is that he wants to be declared disabled."

Bingo, Doug just synthesized our forty-five-minute interview.

Dr. Jones focuses on the disability angle, talking with Doug about what diagnoses could yield a disability classification. "No physical issue here for disability, right?" Dr. Jones inquires.

Doug nods, "My exam was normal."

"Tell me more about his risk taking," Dr. Jones says.

I stand in the corner, silent and amazed at Doug's ability to condense the complexities of his interview with Joe into a three-minute summary.

Rubbing his chin, Dr. Jones summarizes, "Can't hold a job, trouble with relationships, grandiose. Who can possibly smoke a carton a day? You'd have to be smoking two at a time." He shakes his head. "You know, Joe's young enough that this could be schizophrenia or a personality disorder. I wonder if he's hearing voices."

"Didn't ask that," Doug fingers his pen, disappointed with himself.

"Don't be too hard on yourself," Dr. Jones says. "You got a lot of information."

"But Dr. Zink is the one that asked where he lived and that opened up everything else," Doug protests.

"You did fine," Dr. Jones reassures, and we follow him into the exam room.

Sure enough, Joe is hearing voices: little men in the television tell him he's worthless. However, he has no intent or plan to hurt himself or anyone else. Dr. Jones relays his concerns and encourages Joe to see a psychiatrist, telling him to have the receptionist at the front desk arrange an appointment. "You can get disability for something like this," he explains.

Joe's eyes widen.

"Any other questions?" Dr. Jones asks.

"Nope," Joe says. As if he is an arthritic old lady, Joe struggles off the exam table through the door, and into the hall as he thanks us and we say our good-byes.

Back in the physician's office, the three of us discuss the encounter. Dr. Jones admits, "I kind of manipulated Joe into seeing a psychiatrist by saying he could get disability, but I think he really has something. What do you think?" He looks at Doug.

"I haven't done psych yet."

Dr. Jones adds, "Well, sometimes people like Joe do better in a small town. The community takes care of them. Tolerates them."

I glance at Doug, wondering how he feels about this statement. During our drive to the clinic, he disclosed that two nights earlier a middle-aged woman came banging on the door of his trailer about 9 P.M.. She insisted that he was hiding a friend of hers who owed her money. Doug tried to tell her that no one was there but him. However, her yelling and screaming escalated; in desperation Doug called the police. They talked with her, and she left the trailer park. "She's harmless," the officer told Doug. "Gets confused sometimes, but wouldn't hurt a flea." I remind Doug of the incident.

He smiles in recognition, "And I didn't tell you that I saw her at the grocery the next day. She didn't even recognize me." Doug summarizes the story for Dr. Jones.

"The realities of small-town life," Dr. Jones says. "You can't hide like you can in a big city."

Doug's brow is furrowed as he mulls something over then asks, "What made you ask Joe about where he lived? Did you know you were going to get that answer?"

I shook my head. "Just being complete. I wanted the whole picture of his supports."

"And sometimes you are surprised at what you find." Doug says.

I nod. Doug had done a good job with this one, and Dr. Jones was especially comfortable with mental health issues. As a future primary care physician, Doug was fortunate to have a preceptor like Dr. Jones who skillfully integrated mental health and physical health in the care of patients.

"Hey, look out the window," Dr. Jones interjects. Joe is doing wheelies on his mountain bike in the parking lot. He weaves between two parked cars then hikes the front wheel up over the cement parking block and halts to a skid with his left foot.

"You'll see him again," Doug says.

"Yup," Dr. Jones says. "And you are going to be a great physician, Doug."

Our Resources and Challenges

Our Resources and Challenges—Synopsis

GWEN WAGSTROM HALAAS

These are eight very different essays addressing issues of human frailty, professional dedication, technology and change, gaping holes in continuity of care, and challenges in communication—some of the very issues that threaten our national health care system today. Common themes within these essays include meeting a patient's basic human needs, caring for the individual in the context of the community/system, and finding the best way to be professionally accountable. Resources and challenges in health care exist throughout and across communities, states, and nations. Understanding and addressing these resources and challenges may be more effective in rural communities. The issues of addressing complex issues with limited resources in a functional system are often better understood and addressed in the context of a community where there are long term relationships, realities of access to care, and dedication to patient, family, and community.

Distrust of the medical system is an unfortunate reality today. Whether you are a patient who feels powerless in the system of care as a result of confusion, lack of communication, and complexity or whether you are a physician frustrated by an equal sense of powerlessness based on the lack of a functional system, the result is a lack of trust. Lack of trust results in an inability or unwillingness to seek care in a timely fashion.

Dr. Bibey writes of a time when "our bottom line was how our patients fared" ("Inside the Mind of a Modern Country Doc"). I believe we all enter medical school with an altruistic goal, and I also believe that physicians, health care leaders, and government leaders recognize that the system is broken and we need to find a way to get back to that bottom line. In the interest of full disclosure, I was a "chart jockey." In search of equal time, my role was to use my expertise as a physician with health care business education—along with the expertise of a well-educated team—to make decisions about stewarding the resources of a health plan to achieve the best outcomes based on the evidence and ethical principles of decision making. This kind of well-organized, transparent approach is necessary in a large system that pays for the health needs of many hundreds of thousands of individuals and families receiving care from thousands of health care workers in many facilities. Doing the right thing sometimes is simpler in an exam room within a small health care facility in a familiar community setting. The business of health care has become removed from that exam room and that community, and we need to use the lessons learned from managed care and tie them back to the community so how the patients fare is the bottom line.

The student is often the closest to the situation with the clearest view, unencumbered by the information overload and the unmet demands of the day. They can ask the question "Why is this need not being met?" in a way that cuts through the nonsense (Tara Frerks's "The Dressing Change"). Likewise, physicians on the front line of care, such as Dr. Carter, can see a clear, innovative way to prepare staff to deal with emergencies ("A Night in the Life of a Rural Emergency Care Team"), and physicians like Dr. Prasad, confronted by unimaginable tragedy, step into the aftermath and do what they can ("Blog: Rural Mississippi"). In a medical world that has become increasingly complex, addressing the simple issues of changing a dressing or the human reality of preparing for death becomes daunting for patient, caregiver, and provider.

So what are we to do? Wring our hands and wait for the next election of our government representatives and leaders to fix the problem? As physicians, health care providers, patients, families, citizens, and community leaders, we must work together to solve this problem. We all need health care services, and we live in the intersecting worlds—rural, suburban, and urban—of health care services, education, and research. The "blue highways" that connect research institutions to health care delivery in the smallest communities are built for two-way traffic ("Practice-Based Research—'Blue Highways' on the NIH Roadmap"). Those roads bring our brightest and most dedicated young people to the universities for health professions education. They carry our sickest family members to the place where they can receive the best care. We have recently coined the phrase "translational research" to encourage the academic researchers to identify the "blue highways" on their maps so that their discoveries will actually make a difference for the patient in the exam room of the clinic. What about good old communication skills? If we see the physician caring for the needs of a community around the clock with dedication and ingenuity born of limited resources as only the LMD, with the connotation that this is less than adequate, what is the likelihood of developing an interest in receiving the translated message? Or what are the chances that the research will be translatable?

As with Dr. Zink, you need to have a connection to have a "place to start the conversation" ("Thank God for My Ass"). "Today we have options," but tomorrow is coming and our health care system is as frail and neglected as Mr. Olson ("Everyone Did Their Part, But"). But there is always hope. It is best seen in many rural communities where health care facilities are often connected under one roof—the clinic, the hospital, and the nursing home. That combination isn't just to save on building costs. It is about human connections and the quality of care that comes from working together with a common purpose. It is about including the patient and their families as members of the team. For those of us without a stable, like Dr. Zink, we can't always rely on someone else's ass to make things right. Unless we work together and consider a patient's needs as more than strictly medical, the complex reality of keeping a community healthy will be fragmented and focused.

These essays are written from visceral memories—situations that evoked an emotional, gut-based response that was unforgettable. When decisions are made by government, health plans, hospitals, or clinics based on a bottom line that does not take into consideration this gut check, the results miss the target. We do need more "humanistic care" and a "saner health insurance system." We also need to have patients and families more engaged with their care, physicians and other care providers who can communicate with and on behalf of patients, and researchers who are connected with communities, physicians, and patients from the beginning so that discovery becomes part of everyday practice. We also need to provide the role models for this needed change to the students who will become the future health care system. The hoped for result would be happier and healthier patients, families, physicians, and communities. Instead of "Everyone Did Their Part, But" we would have "Everyone Did Their Part, And."

Everyone Did Their Part, But

THERESE ZINK

Late in the afternoon, the effects of my midafternoon cup of coffee were dwindling. I picked up the chart of a new patient with the chief complaint, "Needs a home health nurse." He sounded like a good patient for Melissa, the nurse-practitioner student who was working with me, to see and sort through the concerns. In the meantime, I saw two other patients.

Melissa emerged from the exam room. "You better sit down for this one."

"Be as concise as you can," I said as calmly as I could.

The patient, eighty-seven years old, had not seen a doctor for twenty-five years. Retired from farming, Mr. Gains and his wife lived alone in a farmhouse outside of town. Their son worked the land, and their daughter ran the dry cleaning store in town, just minutes away. The daughter said she cared for them twenty-four hours a day, made their meals, bathed them, everything. It was getting to be too much. Two days ago, her father quit walking and eating. Her mother used a walker. They needed someone to come in and help.

Melissa and I entered the exam room. The daughter, a middle-aged bottle blonde, who was generous with her makeup, rose from her chair. I introduced myself and told her that Melissa had filled me in. "What's your main concern?" I asked.

"It's getting to be too much. I need some help. I thought maybe a nurse once a week," she said as she moved toward the door.

Mr. Gains was frail, wearing a feed cap and overalls. When I addressed him, he made eye contact but didn't say much. We learned that he spent most of the day in a reclining chair, that he was usually incontinent at night. He never had much of an appetite. Both the daughter and son checked on the couple throughout the day.

"Dad doesn't have insurance, so my brother doesn't want much done," the daughter said tapping her toe on the linoleum floor.

"But he's over sixty-five. He should have Medicare," I said.

"Neither of my parents have it."

Strange, I thought, and asked the daughter to step out of the room while Melissa and I did an exam. She was reluctant to do so, so I walked her down the hall and reassured her that we would bring her in as soon as we were done. "Please, they don't have much money," she told me.

I reiterated that we would do the best we could.

When I returned to the room, Melissa had helped Mr. Gains onto the exam table, which was low to the floor, making it easier for elderly patients.

"Pretty unsteady on your feet, aren't you Mr. Gains," Melissa said.

"Do you hurt anywhere?" I asked.

Mr. Gains shook his head.

I asked the usual questions about vomiting, fever, chills, diarrhea. . . . Mr. Gains denied all. Finally, I inquired, "Is anyone hurting you?"

Again, Mr. Gains shook his head. As we removed his flannel shirt, I noticed a layer of brown oily scum around his neck and under his arms. His odor was pungent, not like urine, but similar to that of overripe fruit. His T-shirt was gray. His lungs were clear, and his heart rhythm was regular. No murmurs. We removed his overalls; they were clean, as were his undershorts. The brown scum was also accumulated at his beltline and in his groin. Melissa removed his threadbare socks. Near his ankles were two quarter-sized bedsores.

"Oh, Mr. Gains, those must hurt," Melissa said. "Maybe he's sitting in the recliner like this." She posed in a semifetal position.

I repeated. "Are these hurting you, Mr. Gains?"

He smiled.

He had no bruises. His vitals signs were stable, no fever. We'd need to get a urine sample and some blood. "Can you urinate for us? Pee?" I asked.

He stared at me.

I repeated it again more slowly and looked at him directly.

"Just went," he said. The daughter wasn't going to wait for him to drink water and give us another sample.

I left him on the exam table with Melissa and went to find a nurse to catheterize him and then to talk with his daughter.

She was at the far corner of the waiting room staring out the window at the parking lot. I asked her to follow me into my office. "He's pretty sick. We'll need to check some blood and catheterize him for a urine sample."

The daughter bit at her thumbnail and nodded.

I told her about the bedsores on his ankles. When she said that she had just noticed them, I didn't remark that they'd been there for a while. "I am worried about you being able to care for him at home. I think we should put him in the hospital for a few days."

"Can he come home tomorrow?"

"I doubt it," I said.

"I'll need to ask my brother," she said abruptly. I showed her the phone.

Mr. Gains was difficult to catheterize, but one of the experienced nurses was successful. His urine looked like milky coffee. Infection, this would be our reason to hospitalize him. Then we could get a social service consult, sort through the lack of Medicare, and see if he belonged at home. I was worried about neglect but decided not to broach this. The daughter was mistrustful enough.

I talked with the admitting physician at the hospital thirty minutes away. They'd closed the hospital in town about ten years ago when the clinic was bought by a hospital system. Now, internists from the clinics rotated as hospitalists. Dr. Jones, who worked at our clinic, was on duty for the week. I decided to send Mr. Gains by ambulance. If the brother did not agree to allow us to hospitalize his father, then I'd push the neglect issue and hospitalize him anyway. Knowing that would only antagonize the family, I wanted to avoid it. I pulled Melissa aside and explained my plan. She was relieved.

Luckily, the brother agreed to the hospitalization. "But only for a few days," the daughter told us.

"We'll do what we can," I said. I asked the nurse to call the ambulance and wrote admitting orders in the electronic medical record, pushed the save button, and then clicked send. The mouse had released a human into the maze.

Indeed, Mr. Gains had a urinary tract infection, probably from his enlarged prostate. The hospital social worker learned that the family had never applied for Social Security or Medicare because they were distrustful of the government. Now to apply, they would be required to pay a penalty—several hundred dollars a month for every month past sixty-five years, over twenty years. If they qualified for Medicaid, then Medicaid would pay the penalty, but that probably meant selling all assets; the farm the son worked was at risk. The way out of this maze was bound to be complicated, with many false starts and dead ends.

Later in the week, when Dr. Jones was back in the office, I asked about Mr. Gains.

"He seems afraid of his daughter. And did you realize he's deaf?"

I knew he was hard of hearing but had not noticed that he was lip reading.

"He's a good lip reader," she said. "We used an interpreter to further investigate the neglect. Mr. Gains signs, but he was very evasive. He did admit that he and his wife are home alone most of the day."

"I am not surprised, those bed sores on his legs."

"We'll do what we can, but the daughter is pushing to get him home."

I asked if anyone had checked on his wife, now home by herself.

"Not yet. The social worker is filing a case with adult protective services in order to get someone into the house."

The next day, I saw that Mr. Gains was on my schedule for the following week. He'd been discharged; the daughter had succeeded. But next week arrived, and Mr. Gains had been removed from my schedule. Memories of Mr. Gains gnawed at me; here was this independent farmer, now vulnerable. Would the system and community agencies serve him well? I asked Dr. Jones about him the next time I saw her.

"Back in the hospital," she said, shaking her head. "Public health did not go out, some screwup, so the social worker called the local police to check what was going on." The long and short of it was that the couple was all alone. Mr. Gains had not been out of his chair in two days, his urinal was filled to the brim and his trousers were wet. His wife was hobbling around with her walker. She said caring for her husband was too much. So the police took Mr. Gains back to the hospital, and he was admitted through the ER. They did X-rays and found that he had an upper arm fracture and that his left hip had disintegrated.

My heart thumped. Melissa, who'd joined the conversation, stared wide eyed. "Did we miss that?"

"We walked him at the hospital, and he did fine, but the hip has clearly been deteriorating for a while," Dr. Jones said.

"I helped him scoot up on the exam table when he was here initially, maybe I caused the arm," Melissa mused.

I felt guilty for not ordering X-rays on the initial admission. If we'd picked it up earlier, would things be different? The gnawing in my gut had been well placed.

"But it gets worse," Dr. Jones said. "Another internist cleared him for surgery and ortho did a total hip replacement. The only way he could be independent was to fix the hip, they said. I was not on duty."

"I'm surprised that he was cleared for surgery," I said aghast.

"Well, he shouldn't have been. Shortly after surgery he had an MI and a blood clot in his lung."

The three of us shook our heads in disbelief. This was a nightmare. An independent farmer was now powerless in the system with no one advocating for him. What did the family think now? They were at the mercy of the health care maze they distrusted.

"We had to make him safe and treat the initial infection," Melissa said. "Everyone was just doing their part."

This was true. Suspicious of neglect, we realized that a home health nurse was not enough and admitted him to the hospital. The social worker investigated. Dr. Jones tried to keep him in the hospital and advised nursing home placement. When he was brought to the ER, the physician ordered X-rays and found the hip and shoulder fractures. The orthopedist repaired the hip so Mr. Gains could be independent. But somehow the pieces did not fit together.

In the old days, the local doctor would have been the one caring for him in the hospital, and given the low-tech approach to treating frail, elderly patients,

Mr. Gains probably would not have had the surgery. But then he probably could not have returned home, either. Today's high-tech medicine means that there are many more players, and if a patient is unable to voice his needs and does not have an advocate, then there are no guarantees. The human gets lost in the maze.

Complicating every step is the family's distrust of the health care system. Because of Mr. Gains's independence, he had not signed up for the government supports to help the elderly. His health problems smoldered because he hadn't seen a doctor in twenty-five years. He had not received the needed care from his children, nor were they acting as his advocates. They wanted him to stay on the farm. No question, this was neglect. But once he had entered the maze, there was a momentum that did not serve him well.

A few days later, one of the long-time clinic nurses handed me an obituary from the previous day. "Thought you'd want to see this."

Mr. Gains had died. I shared it with Melissa who said, "Now he's at peace." I told the nurse and Melissa that I thought we should go to the viewing or funeral, but that the family probably wanted nothing to do with us.

The nurse asked me if I knew where they lived.

I shook my head.

"You should drive by. It will put everything in perspective." She gave me the address and directions.

The next day, I drove out to the farm. It took me an hour to locate the right gravel road. I tried to diffuse my frustration with deep breaths and enjoy the scenery. Fields separated by fences and distinguished by the direction of the planted rows rolled out like a patchwork quilt, stretching to the horizon in every direction. The land of big sky, today it was cornflower blue and cloudless. Corn and soybean fields were half harvested and dotted with farm equipment that looked like toys from the distance. I passed two farmers in their colossal tractors on the road, large clumps of earth left in their wake.

At the junction of two gravel roads, the Gains's house sat in a stand of mature oaks. You could tell the two-story white clapboard house was lovely in its day, but it had been thirsty for paint for at least a decade. Tattered blinds hung in the upstairs window. Rusting cars and farm implements were parked in a patch of weed trees. One of the out buildings had collapsed. A beautiful spot, once upon a time, but like the Gainses it had aged. I realized how isolated the Gainses were because they didn't drive. In this small community, where everyone knows everyone's business, no one had come forward about their situation. The invisible rules of silence, not interfering.

I clocked the mileage back to town—six miles, half of which was on gravel roads. More than the "few minutes" the daughter had described.

This piece was published in the February 2008 issue of *Minnesota Medicine*.

Inside the Mind of a Modern Country Doc

TOM BIBEY

I have seen a lot of changes in my three decades of practice. Technological advancement offers new treatments, and I am grateful for them. Heck, I have partaken of this myself. Last fall I had a retinal detachment, and with modern ophthalmology I was back to 20/20 in no time. Don't get me wrong, I've nothing against being modern.

Computers have improved our ability to compile data, but also have rendered privacy obsolete. Sure, I know the Government enacted the HIPAA privacy rules, but that was only to keep everyone else from cutting in on their business. Look at it this way: HIPAA was enacted by the same crowd who invented the Social Security number. I don't know about you, but that scares me a bit.

As a small businessman for years, I know the importance of the bottom line. Years ago, the staff and I agonized about increasing office visits from fifteen to seventeen dollars. We were very concerned as to how a two-dollar increase might play in the local circles. My aunt would hear about it and talk bad about me in Sunday school. In small towns, you have to be careful about a bad PR rep at church or in the beauty shops. A local restaurant owner who got greedy and went up a full dollar on a perch plate was out of business in a month. When you live with people, your decisions tend to be conservative, and we were sensitive to local economic issues.

Our bottom line was how our patients fared. If they were happy, and we cleared enough to go another year, we counted it a success. It was like one of my patients said, "I want you to make enough to retire, Doc, just not in a few years." I agreed and found it good counsel.

Somewhere along the way, medicine evolved into big business. Once the bottom line became a stockholder report, the rules began to change. An old doc, Dr. William Gray, had the same answer for every problem. "I don't know what's wrong here, but it's got something to do with money." Well, old Doc is long gone, but I think he's still right.

In the early 1980s, I made almost all my decisions in conjunction with my patient, together with the specialists we deemed appropriate in a given case.

It wasn't but a few years before modern medical "oversight" or "management" began to assert itself. This started first with government programs, soon followed by big business. Docs were forced to learn a new set of skills to overcome these obstacles to the delivery of care.

Early on, it was a benign process. Every once in a while I'd get a call from old Doc Smith who'd ask about a case. I knew him from State Medical Society meetings. Retired, he'd never made all that much when he was in practice, so I understood his need to supplement his income. I'd even taken over some of his patients, so Doc Smith knew me well. He wasn't going to scoop me on much over the phone. I had the advantage of being the doc who saw the patient, and we both knew he wasn't in a position to compete with that. Doc had to call every so often. I understood. He'd call and ask a few questions, and I'd tell him in doctor terms about where to go, and we'd laugh.

By the mideighties the minor nuisance grew to a downright disruption of patient care. I remember a fellow I had followed since I started my practice. I inherited him when a local doc retired. The patient was elderly and had multiple medical problems: several heart attacks, a pacemaker revised several times, bad kidneys, bad lungs, but he was a heck of a nice guy.

My first hospital admission for the patient was for an episode of syncope (they call it "falling out" around here) and the situation was complex, so an extensive workup was undertaken. Both carotid arteries had partial blockage, but the surgeon said that the literature showed that only the worst side of a 70 percent blockage warranted intervention. (Here is a country doc tip for you: if a surgeon doesn't want to operate, I would take that advice very seriously.) I talked it over with the local cardiologist, we ran everything by the big boys at the Medical Center, and everyone agreed to a treatment plan. With some adjustments in medication, we sent the patient home. Surgery, at least at that time, was not indicated. A week later, he had an unanticipated TIA (near ministroke), which thankfully resolved. Due to the change in circumstances, the surgeons changed their minds and proceeded with surgery to correct his right carotid artery blockage. The patient did well, and he went home satisfied with the outcome. For him, it was the end of that chapter of his story. For me it was the beginning.

Six weeks later, I got a letter from one of the Medicare review boys, who determined the first admission to be unnecessary. I knew my patient could get stuck with the tab, so I began to compose a letter of explanation. Before I could complete it, I had a second letter on my desk from a different review bureaucrat (I call them chart jockeys). This jockey determined the second hospital stay was due to a premature discharge from the first admission. I have a fair amount of education, but I was confused. How can one be discharged too early from an unnecessary admission?

I found it a silly demonstration of the lack of medical sophistication on the part of the reviewers, but I did not anticipate the intense effort required to win this battle. However, I lost the war. Years later I noticed reviewer number one had his name on a government medical complex, and I assure you I will labor in obscurity until the end. I'll consider myself lucky if I just stay out of trouble. I was the doc for my patient until the end, when he died of plain old, very old, age. Every so often we delighted in laughing at the incompetence of those chart jockeys.

During the next decade, the battle of the hospital bureaucrats reached full-pitched intensity, and we country docs fought on the front lines all alone for our hospitalized patients. This was one reason I later quit hospital work; it was too time consuming to fight on two simultaneous fronts. Now, I am thankful we have hospitalists to help with this onslaught. If a patient had a serum sodium of 120, regardless of how bad they felt, or if they were dehydrated from diarrhea, it would not justify admission, yet if the same parameter were less than 130 on the day of discharge, and the patient had any problem arise in the next thirty-one days that required admission, it would be deemed "poor quality of care." I never understood that. Either your sodium is low and you need to spend a night in a hospital or you don't, and no one from the government ever explained it to me.

Things deteriorated in the 1990s with the alphabet soup. COLA, CLIA, OSHA, HIPAA, EMTALA. I've heard the powers that be are going to start up the NBEMAA (National Bureau for the Elimination of Medical Abbreviations Agency) to question everyone's integrity for use of nongovernment approved abbreviations. Now if they do, I guess I'm gonna call it a day. The hypocrisy would just be too much.

Over the ensuing decade, I did learn how to circumvent EMTALA (Emergency Medical Treatment and Active Labor Act). I call it "the EMTALA end run." If by chance a doc has a patient who wound up in the wrong facility and can't find anyone to accept a transfer, you do "the EMTALA end run": tell the family to check the patient out AMA (Against Medical Advice—I try not to use abbreviations). Arrange for an ambulance to take the patient to a facility that has the specialist they need, such as neurology or cardiac surgery. Once there, the family can demand their loved one receive the specialized care not available at the first institution. This is an insider country doc trick, and it works every time.

Oversight of medicines would be even more humorous, if not so sad. One elderly patient came to see me and complained of being weak, nervous, and dizzy. Being the smart doc I was, I figured the three diuretics she was taking had something to do with it, so I changed her regimen to one that reflected current clinical rationale. In short order, she spun out of control, and became incoherent and combative. She was hospitalized for an intensive evaluation, only to find the resolution to the problem to be the urgent reinstitution of her old regimen. She returned to normal in a few days and again was weak, nervous, and dizzy. I knew the chart jockeys would come around in six weeks, and no one would understand, so I arranged a nephrology consult. (This guy was one of the smartest docs on our staff—the cats that get acid/base are always quick.)

I'll never forget the nephrologist's thorough review of the entire medical record, and that poor woman doing her best to answer all those questions again. In the end, he told me it made no scientific sense, but he would continue her antiquated regimen. We all do our duty, I guess. I am still the patient's doc; the patient is still weak, nervous, and dizzy; the nephrologist left town for a big-city practice where he can make some real money; and the chart jockeys still send letters. Some things never change, and all these government folks who believe they can morph these country people via legislation are naive as to medicine and human behavior.

By 2000, we had all the best new technology. X-ray is instant access. I have a palm pilot that catalogs every drug interaction known to man, which I consult every hour of the day. The EMR has a complete medical record on each patient, at least for anything done in our system. At the same time, this open access has made it a field day for all sorts of armchair amateurs trying to cut costs and improve quality. On a good day, they are a nuisance. On a bad one, the meddling is dangerous. Take it from an old doc; it is still true to this modern day—if you don't know the patient, you don't know anything.

The insurance companies love to play doctor. Take my noncompliant diabetic patient with a hemoglobin A1C that does not meet goal. The first order of business, since I wish to stay in practice, is to send him to an endocrinologist. If possible, one should bolster the case by the choice of one from a medical center. A year later, the patient will still have the same numbers, unless he comes to Jesus and decides to change his life. The cost of the endocrinologist changed nothing but increased the bill to insurance, and my risk as a target for the blame is dramatically lowered due to the referral.

Then there is the daily war of which medications are on the insurance company formulary—don't get me started. The company knows what it's doing. It is a sick game, but $34 million a year later, I'm certain the insurance CEO doesn't care. The patients can't get a straight answer from the insurance crowd, so they wind up in our office angry with us for not being able to get their medicine. Sometimes it is a heck of way to spend your day.

I don't know where all this is headed, but I have concerns. A few of my patients were dropped from insurance plans due to their failure to comply with some company regulation. I suspect with growth of the database, the insurance companies will be able to identify outliers (more expensive patients) with increased accuracy. I'm afraid this will be used as an excuse to exclude any patient who is projected not to generate an adequate profit. Well, I am not enthusiastic about the prospect of insurance company decisions as to who is worth what.

Ever wonder what directs the daily scooter traffic? Like many docs, I have had patients walk in demanding a form be completed so they can get a free power scooter, only to walk out angry when I "wouldn't fill out the form right." This almost always generates a letter from the scooter salespeople who highlight the lines on the form I need to change so the patient can get his or her scooter. Many of these patients will get it approved elsewhere. I used to call the Medicare hotline to complain and received a few forms to fill out, but that was the end of it. I suspect the power scooter lobby is stronger in Washington than the country doctor lobby. In my case, it would have to be, 'cause the only time I have been up there is to show the kids the Smithsonian and the Declaration of Independence. I don't know what drives a man to be the best scooter salesman he can, but my guess is it has to do with the fact he can make more money in the Medicare scooter business than by the sophisticated eye surgery my ophthalmologist did when he saved my eye last fall.

I reckon old Doc Gray was about right. On all these issues, I don't know what went wrong here, but it's got something to do with money. How the bottom line has changed; I no longer worry about two dollar office visit increases. Nowadays my aunt isn't worried about it either. She's more concerned that my uncle has cancer and can't get his medications approved. He is approaching his lifetime limit, and his secondary won't pay on anything Medicare deems unnecessary. She spends more and more time with the paperwork and would prefer tending to Uncle Fred instead of anonymous government or insurance employees.

It's 2008. I've come a long way, baby. Now I am in a daily fight to get my patients the care they need. I'd rather spend my time with my patients, but I've had to adapt to offer any care at all. Over time, my strategy has become finely tuned, and I don't have quite as much trouble with the insurance chart jockeys as I used to. In a way, I hate to let any outsiders in on it, because I have a few more years I want to practice, and I hate to tip my hand to the enemy. I suppose I will as long as you promise to share this last segment with working docs only.

I agree that most high-tech radiographic studies are a waste of time and money, not to mention unneeded radiation. In this consumer-driven world, I'd bet a full third are unnecessary, but there is little way out. If it is demanded and has the remotest possibility of being diagnostic, and if you don't give in . . . well, let me put it this way: I have to have malpractice insurance to go to work every day.

When you need a high-tech study and the health insurance company won't give in, here's how to work the system. Again, this is a proven method, Dr. Bibey tested, and a virtual foolproof plan. Not long ago, I had a patient in a car wreck.

He went to the ER and had a negative plain C-spine film. A few days later he was in my office, still complaining of neck pain, but now with radiculopathy. (Pain down the arm.) That did it. I wanted an MRI.

The insurance company nurse would not approve the study because the patient had not completed her protocol of the completion of two anti-inflammatory medications and physical therapy. The game was on.

Again, I am more than aware that too many fancy studies are done in this world, but post-trauma neck pain with radiculopathy? The review nurse wouldn't budge, which left me to do battle with the physician medical cost overseer. I had to wait for an appointment.

They gave me a phone appointment in an hour or so. I held as the company "elevator music" droned. Lord, at least they could come up with some hip music. A recorded message stated the call would be monitored for quality assurance purposes, an indication you might get a person before too long. After a long wait, someone came to the phone. He was most cordial but assured me the test was not needed and, like the nurse, was not moved by any concerns for my patient. It was time to pull out the big guns.

He was a physician, so I decided to appeal to that. I do not like to ingratiate myself to these kinds of doctors, but it was a calculated move. It seemed the means justified the ends.

"Doc, if you would, how 'bout turning off that recorder. Let's talk doctor to doctor." I was pleasant, but I had that luxury. I knew where this was going.

"We usually don't do that."

"Well, I don't want to get you in any trouble, so I wish you would. I need to ask a question."

There was a click. "Done."

"Look pal, I've been around this business a long time, and I care about these patients. I don't know why I keep doing it, I guess I make a third of what you do, if that. Think you could get me a job?"

"Perhaps. I can refer you to HR."

"Hm. Might do that. You like working there?"

"Yes, it is excellent. No call. Good salary and benefits. Home every night. I recommend it highly."

"I see. Oh, let me tell you something about this patient. His uncle is the meanest badass plaintiff's attorney in Virginia. He does some cases around these parts. Martin Taylor is the name. He handled one of these a few years ago—very similar circumstances—bad outcome. The retail price for the injury was about eight million. In case this one goes bad too, all I need to know is what percentage you plan to pay, 'cause I ain't gonna give a dime. I don't think my boss will want to contribute either, but I'll call him as soon as we hang up. I doubt you can count on your corporate boys—loyalty is mighty slim nowadays in this business. I'm sure you understand."

There was silence for a moment, then a click. The recorder was back on. "Let's see, Dr. Bibey. That MRI accession number is "A" as in apple, then 45B as in boy. . ." And so it went.

"Thank you, sir, and have a good day."

And therein lies the practical lesson for the day. There are two kinds of people in health care. Eighty percent are those who do right because that is in their nature and because they want to. The other 20 percent, like this gentleman, have to be positioned to see it is in their best interest to do so. They are often the highest paid ones, so it takes some work, but they'll come around with enough pressure. None of these business guys go to church with the people they impact, so it makes no difference to them. All you gotta do is figure out how the age-old human weaknesses of greed and money figure into the equation, and then push the buttons.

Well, I find it a shame it had to come to all that. All I wanted was to be a good doc and care for my patients with compassion. Instead, the system has forced me to be a savvy street fighter just to see another day in the ring. I would have preferred to spend my adult life immersed in medical studies and in discussion of odd cases in doctors' lounge conversations. I wish my business acumen could have been confined to the skills of a young doc who worried how his aunt might think of him if he went up two full dollars on an office visit. It wasn't to be. Instead, I was forced to dream up survival strategies for both me and for my patients.

Still, I wouldn't change places with the chart jockeys or anyone else. I got to read plenty of doctor books for fun, and most important, at least I had the honor to be a doc. Sir William Osler, the father of modern medicine, said, "Seeing patients without reading books is like going to sea without a compass, but reading books without seeing patients is like not going to sea at all." I'd rather be the cat who sees the patients than the one who issues all those silly edicts and pronouncements. I would not trade places with the executive who takes home thirty mil' a year, even if what I do is not as prestigious and sure doesn't pay as well.

I guess it is like what Lee Trevino said about golf. When he hit the senior tour, someone interviewed him and was struck by the absence of trophies on the mantle.

"Where are all your trophies?" the reporter asked.

"Don't need 'em." Trevino replied. "I know what I've done."

I'm not sure what the chart jockey, some bored bureaucrat, or the health care business executive will believe in the end, but as for me, like Lee Trevino, I know what I've done too. Like brother Lee, I got to play the real game, and played for the sheer love of it. I got to be Doc, and I wouldn't trade the experience for any material gain.

Practice-Based Research—"Blue Highways" on the NIH Roadmap

JOHN M. WESTFALL, JAMES MOLD, AND LYLE FAGNAN

On the old highway maps of America, the main routes were red, and the back roads blue. Now even the colors are changing. But in those brevities just before dawn and a little after dusk—times neither day nor night—the old roads return to the sky some of its color. Then, in truth, they carry a mysterious cast of blue, and it's that time when the pull of the blue highway is strongest, when the open road is a beckoning, a strangeness, a place where a man can lose himself.

William Least Heat-Moon, *Blue Highways*

U.S. 34 drops out of the Rockies like so many spring-fed creeks. Passing through the front-range sprawl of bedroom communities and suburbs, it narrows to two lanes and begins its trek across the Great Plains. In its heyday it was a bustling highway with countless travelers from the East Coast and Midwest on their way to vacation in the cool Colorado mountains. Now it lies still, a blue highway, heat rising in waves off the pavement, dotted with small, dusty farming communities. A promise on one hometown brochure proudly states, "Just an hour from I-70."

But don't be fooled. The communities through which it runs are active, vital centers of business and agriculture. A lot of life happens in these communities, and a lot of health care is delivered. The "blue highways" connect these small, vital communities to the roaring interstate system, linking people, commerce, and ideas across our vast country. Even though most Americans do not live in rural towns, the majority live in communities far removed from the academic tertiary medical centers where most federally funded research is conducted, and it's not only distance that separates these two worlds.

The National Institutes of Health (NIH) spend billions of dollars annually on biomedical research. Most of this money is spent on basic research that aims to understand how living organisms work. A relatively smaller but increasing amount is spent on clinical studies involving people. A new initiative called the "NIH Roadmap" has focused increased attention on the need to "translate" basic research into human studies and then, hopefully, into information that can improve clinical practice and ultimately benefit patients.[1] The NIH Roadmap may benefit from the "blue highway" research that connects the major academic science laboratories to the physicians and patients in primary care offices across the United States.

Inventing a new medicine or treatment is only the starting point for improving the health of an individual patient. The magnitude and nature of the work required to translate findings from human medical research into valid and effective clinical practice have been underestimated. Frequently, years or even decades are required. It takes an estimated average of seventeen years for only 14 percent of new scientific discoveries to enter day-to-day clinical practice.[2] Americans receive only 50 percent of the recommended preventive, acute, and long-term health care.[3] For example, although colon cancer screening is well studied, only half of eligible Americans have received the appropriate screening.[4]

Myriad detours, speed traps, roadblocks, and potholes limit the movement of treatments from bench to practice. They include the limited external validity of randomized controlled trials, the diverse nature of primary care office practice, the paucity of successful collaborative efforts between academic researchers and community physicians and patients, and the failure of the academic research enterprise to address needs indentified by the community.[5]

The vast majority of patients receive medical care in the primary care office setting, yet the majority of clinical research occurs in the academic clinic setting.[6] Clinical research studies, with their tight inclusion and exclusion criteria, create an artificial sample of patients who do not represent the majority of those who present to primary care offices across the United States. Because treatment recommendations and disease management guidelines are often based on evidence from a relatively small number of large tertiary care centers, their applicability to the everyday practice of medicine may be limited. A guideline on managing upper respiratory infections, based on evidence and derived by an expert panel through consensus, was found to be a failure because only 13 percent of the patients with cold symptoms who came into their doctors' offices were actually eligible for the care outlined in the guideline.[7] The majority had other health issues that disqualified them. Frequently, the major questions that need to be answered to close the gaps between scientific discovery and widespread use in primary care are not prioritized by funders or undertaken by academic researchers. For example, there are many studies about hypertension, and hypertension treatment guidelines are routinely updated and distributed. Yet fundamental questions are unresolved. What is the benefit to lowering blood pressure an additional 10 mm Hg by adding another medicine (for example from 130/90 to 130/80)? Patients want to know if the benefit is worth the costs of taking yet another pill.

Essential elements in the NIH Roadmap are the translational steps; translation of basic science laboratory work in animals into basic human medical chemistry and physiology, translation of basic human chemistry and physiology into improved diagnostic tests, medicine, and treatments for use in clinical practice. The final crucial step in clinical care is the delivery of recommended care to the right patient at the right time, resulting in the improvement in that patient's health.

Missing from the NIH Roadmap are the "blue highways" that form a two-way connection between the interstates of academic scientific discoveries and the patients receiving care in the primary care office setting. Without translation to office practice, individual patient care will not change.

A potential solution to these problems is the expansion of "practice-based research," research that is grounded in, informed by, and intended to improve clinical practice. Practice-based research occurs in the office, where most patients receive most of their care most of the time and may be the essential link between bench discoveries, bedside efficacy, and everyday clinical effectiveness. Physicians in an office agree to join a network of other offices to participate in studies. Office staff is involved in assisting study staff enroll patients and collect the data. The study questions that can be examined in this manner look at the day-to-day problems that present in primary care office practice. Practice-based research is the best setting for studying the process of care and the manner in which diseases are diagnosed, treatments initiated, and chronic conditions managed. It is in practice-based research networks where effectiveness can be measured, where new clinical questions may arise, where readiness to change and adopt new treatments can be studied and addressed, where patient knowledge and preferences are encountered and managed, and where the interface between a patient and doctor can be explored and medical care improved.[8]

Practice-based research has a long and robust history in the United States and throughout the world but receives limited attention from mainstream academic clinical research laboratories and the NIH.[9] With the leadership of the Agency of Healthcare Research and Quality, more than one hundred networks are funded and actively conducting practice-based research across the United States.[10]

Without the "blue highways" of practice-based research, we are concerned that the NIH Roadmap will simply transport research ideas back and forth between the academic tertiary and quaternary care centers. Biomedical discoveries may never make it past the academic medical center, and the unanswered questions of day-to-day clinical care may never be addressed by the scientific community. The two-way interface between clinical practice and scientific laboratory must be reimagined and strengthened. The best new treatments will achieve little if they never reach the patients for whom they were developed.

The physicians engaged in practice-based research are eager to conduct research that will help bring those discoveries to their patients. However, practice-based research is more than a conduit to patients. Practice-based research provides the laboratory that will help generate new knowledge and bridge the chasm between recommended care and improved health. Slowing down for the old "two-lane highway" may actually bring more science to the majority of Americans.

Just as "blue highway" has entered the American travel lexicon, our hope is that "practice-based research" will enter the mainstream medical research vocabulary and become a strong component of the NIH Roadmap. Practice-based research is a crucial scientific step, the "blue highway," between the great medical advances of the next twenty-five years and the millions of Americans who want to live long and healthy lives.

NOTES

Heat-Moon, William Least. *A Journey into America: Blue Highways.* Boston: Back Bay Books, 1999.

1. Zerhouni, Elias. "The NIH Roadmap." *Science* 302.5642 (2003): 63–72.

2. Balas, E. Andrew, and Suzanne. A. Boren. "Managing Clinical Knowledge for Health Care Improvement." *Yearbook of Medical Informatics.* Stuttgart, German: Schattauer Verlagsgesellschaft, 2000.

3. McGlynn, Elizabeth A., Steven M. Asch, John Adams et al. "The Quality of Health Care Delivered to Adults in the United States." *New England Journal of Medicine* 348 (2003): 2635–45.

4. Coughlin, Steven S., and Trevor D. Thompson. "Colorectal Cancer Screening Practices among Men and Women in Rural and Nonrural Areas of the United States, 1999," *Journal of Rural Health* 20.2 (2004): 118–24.

5. Sung, Nancy S., William F. Crowley Jr., Myron Genel et al. "Central Challenges Facing the National Clinical Research Enterprise." *Journal of American Medical Association* 289.10 (2003): 1278–87.

6. White, Kerr L., T. Franklin Williams, and Bernard G. Greenberg. "The Ecology of Medical Care." *New England Journal of Medicine* 265 (1961): 885–92; Green, Larry A., George E. Fryer Jr., Barbara. P. Yawn et al. "The Ecology of Medical Care Revisited." *New England Journal of Medicine* 344.26 (2001): 2021–25.

7. O'Connor, Patrick J., Gayle Amundson, and John Christianson. "Performance Failure of an Evidence-Based Upper Respiratory Infection Clinical Guideline." *Journal of Family Practice* 48.9 (1999): 690–97.

8. Westfall, John M., Rebecca F. Van Vorst, Joe McGloin et al. "Triage and Diagnosis of Chest Pain in Rural Hospitals: Implementation of the ACI-TIPI in the High Plains Research Network." *Annals of Family Medicine* 4.2 (2006): 153–58; Main, Deborah S., Lawrence J. Lutz, James E. Barrett et al. "The Role of Primary Care Clinician Attitudes, Beliefs, and Training in the Diagnosis and Treatment of Depression." *Archives of Family Medicine* 2.10 (1993): 1061–66; Taylor, James A., Tao Sheng Kwan-Gett, and Edward M. McMahon Jr. "Effectiveness of a Parental Educational Intervention in Reducing Antibiotic Use in Children: A Randomized Controlled Trial." *Pediatric Infectious Disease Journal* 24.6 (2005): 489–93; Stange, Kurt C., Susan A. Flocke, Meredith A. Goodwin et al. "Direct Observation of Rates of Preventive Service Delivery in Community Family Practice." *Preventive Medicine* 31.2 (2000): 167–76.

9. Green, Larry A., and John Hickner. "A Short History of Primary Care Practice-Based Research Networks: From Concept to Essential Research Laboratories." *Journal of the American Board of Family Medicine* 19.1 (2006): 1–10.

10. See the Agency for Healthcare Research and Quality (AHRQ) Web site. With the leadership of the AHRQ, more than one hundred networks are funded and actively conducting practice-based research across the United States.

A longer version of this was published in the *Journal of American Medical Association* 297.4 (2007): 403–6.

Local Medical Doctors: State-of-the-Art Healers

GWEN WAGSTROM HALAAS

In an emergency room in Cambridge, Massachusetts, at Harvard Medical School, I first heard the acronym "LMD." As a medical student, this was one more acronym to add to my brain, already swimming with acronyms and millions of bits of information. I soon realized that LMD was the house staff's term of derision for the local doctors whose patients they were presenting. This was news to me, that other doctors would not respect their peers. Maybe I was naive, coming from Minnesota where we are "all above average." This realization dulled the shiny image of the medical mecca that I had the privilege of experiencing. Moving back to Minneapolis, I managed to escape this attitude for a while, training in a hospital where the family of family doctors was the valued source of patients and referrals. This attitude resurfaced as my peers joined practices in small communities in Minnesota, and I would hear them complain about how they were treated by the urban consultants.

On my rural rotation in Homer, Alaska, I was first introduced to the amazing level of care rendered in a rural setting. While on call one evening in the hospital, a man with chest pain arrived in the emergency room. He was quickly evaluated, treated with streptokinase, stabilized, and put on a Lear jet to Anchorage. This was months before anyone in the big city of Minneapolis was considering thrombolysis for acute MIs (heart attacks). I bragged about this experience and others on my return to the city. They looked at me like I must be hallucinating.

In my professional journey, I first started my own family practice on the skyway downtown—a very old-fashioned general practice in a fancy setting in St. Paul. From there I traveled through combinations of practice, teaching and managing the business of health care until I found myself directing a program that taught medical students the basics of medicine by immersing them in rural community practices. Again face to face with *LMD*s, I marveled at the innovative ways they cared for families and communities. These "hick" towns have helicopters, digital X-rays, telemedicine, electronic health records, robot consultants, medication vending machines, and approaches to care that are on the cutting edge. Their state-of-the-art facilities are patient-centered healing environments.

I learned from students in these communities about surgeons who started providing laparoscopic procedures before their counterparts in the city. These same surgeons set up a state-of-the-art operating room in a third-world setting to provide surgical services and train their local doctors. The students not only get hands-on experience with hundreds of procedures (many times the experience of their urban peers), but they are also exposed to cutting-edge treatment and the commitment to serve others with the technology and training toward sustainable, quality care.

Another physician from one of the program's smallest communities developed the Combined Advanced Life Support (CALS) course to provide the necessary resuscitation skills for providers who are the first contact for any emergency in rural or remote settings. This community has trained many of its health professionals who are the first responders in many statewide disasters. The small hospital has an intensive care room with telemedicine equipment dedicated to rapid response for stroke patients. Patients can be evaluated by a neurological consultant, treated, and transferred within minutes to a tertiary care facility. A nearby helicopter is ready for quick transport for the needed care.

These communities are often able to decide to invest in technology or innovation earlier because of a smaller total investment and a simpler bureaucracy to navigate. Decisions are made to better serve the community, including digital X-rays accessible immediately in the clinic, electronic health records that connect facilities and transmit prescriptions quickly and accurately, or contracting with radiologists on the other side of the world to provide evening X-ray readings. Innovation is born of need.

As a family physician visiting these communities, I envy their practice because of the multilevel-care facilities that are their medical home. The clinic, hospital, nursing home, pharmacy, and emergency or urgent care facility are often all in one. I look back at my own busy practice and dream of how things might have been organized in a more efficient system of care. This efficiency is not just a result of fewer steps but of closer relationships and improved communication and familiarity with the patients, their families, and their community context. The students are quick to appreciate their settings and are often amazed by the depth of relationships and the meaningful familiarity their preceptors have with their patients from years of caring for them. As students, they truly appreciate being a valued member of the team and of the community. Health care staff always think of the students, calling them in to see their most interesting patients and giving them hands-on experience. Community patients take their role in teaching students seriously. Students are greeted in the grocery store by people they have seen in the clinic or hospital and can easily see a future role as a respected and valued caregiver.

These LMDs are dedicated to providing quality health care services to their community. This dedication is not just to their daily work of caring for each patient but to the success of the system as a whole. In addition to their patient care, they pitch in to lead and manage the health care delivery system. They do this as clinic medical directors, hospital chiefs of staff, nursing home medical directors, sports team physicians, and heads of the ambulance service. Family physicians often practice a broad scope of medicine—from clinic to emergency room to hospital to nursing home and to the operating room.

This dedication goes beyond patient care to the community. These LMDs are often civic leaders engaged in developing successful businesses, supporting the education systems, and contributing to music and the arts. They are also committed to the future. Hundreds of Minnesota physicians are products of the rural medical school program and then choose to teach the next generation of physicians who will become their partners.

Where would these communities be without this dedicated service and leadership? Regardless of size, geography, or cultural diversity, the success of these towns—prairie towns, lakeside villages, mining towns, agricultural centers—is often dependent on their health care systems. The individuals who choose to be LMDs are extraordinary and along with their families have invested their lives and energy in their communities. These are the role models we want to train the physicians of the future who will care for us and for our communities.

A Night in the Life of a Rural Emergency Care Team: The Value of the Comprehensive Advanced Life Support Program

DARRELL L. CARTER

Another cold blustery January night in northwestern Minnesota, and you hope everyone stays home and your hospital's emergency department remains quiet. As the night charge nurse on duty, you are responsible for overseeing the care your night staff (one other RN and an LPN) gives to the twelve inpatients in your twenty-two bed Critical Access Hospital (CAH). These twelve patients include a mother and her hours-old newborn and an eighty-two-year-old female who is two days post-op after a hip pinning and who is exhibiting increased confusion and agitation. You hope to let your on-call doctor get some sleep since she was up much of last night delivering the baby in your nursery. The only other practicing physician in your community is gone for a much-deserved five-day break to Cancun.

All has remained routine until 1:00 A.M. when the squawk from your ambulance paging radio disturbs your charting. The Basic Life Support ambulance is dispatched to a motor-vehicle-crash involving two vehicles and an unknown number of victims. At least two of the patients sound seriously injured. Reluctantly, you shift your role from more mundane tasks to organizing the team for the soon-to-be-busy emergency department.

In the twenty-first century, seriously ill or injured patients benefit from a growing amount of advanced technology for diagnosis and treatment of their ailments or injuries. Highly trained specialists are now available to help manage a wide variety of complex conditions, and well-trained and highly skilled teams staff emergency departments. Unfortunately, this is true only in the larger population centers of the United States. Rural health care facilities do not have immediate access to this wide variety of specialists and frequently lack the more advanced equipment needed to diagnose or treat the seriously ill or injured patient. Rural providers frequently lack the organized team, knowledge, and skills to rapidly perform the life-saving procedures and treatments needed by the more seriously ill or injured patients. Extensive distances lengthen the time required to transport patients to specialized urban medical centers for life- or organ-saving procedures. It is little wonder that rural trauma victims have a higher mortality rate than their urban counterparts. In 2004 the Minnesota Statewide Trauma System reported that fewer than 30 percent of all motor vehicle crashes occurred in rural areas, but 70 percent of the fatal crashes are rural.

There are many obstacles to our delivering the highest and most modern emergency and critical care to rural patients. However, the medical legal standards of care and the general public expect similar care to be delivered in both urban and rural communities. Disparity in the availability of advanced emergency care has adverse consequences. In rural areas, these include: higher rates of trauma deaths, increased burnout among providers, difficulty recruiting staff for existing health care facilities, and an increase in medical-legal risks for practitioners due to the inability to rapidly deliver emergency care or obtain easy consultation for some critically ill or injured patients.

So what is the solution to this developing crisis in rural medicine? Some recommend more helicopters to rapidly transport the rural patients to urban centers. Others promote equipping rural communities with all the latest equipment, as well as hiring skilled specialists to respond to the infrequent events. But is society willing to finance the cost of such solutions? Others claim living (and vacationing and driving) in the rural parts of our country is simply more dangerous, so if you elect to live in, or even venture into rural areas, then you need to accept the inherent risks.

Out of a feeling of inadequacy to deal with the wide array of clinical problems and the desire to improve the outcomes of rural patients came the concept that there is a better way to prepare the rural health care team for the variety of medical emergencies that arise. Although traditional advanced life support courses such as Advanced Cardiac Life Support and Advanced Trauma Life Support offer valuable education to thousands of health care providers, they don't meet all of the needs of rural providers. Each course presents an excellent summation of the major treatment protocols for a specific aspect of emergency care such as trauma, cardiac, pediatric, newborn, or obstetric, but they include much overlap of subject matter and fall short in meeting many of the rural provider's needs such as the management of the difficult airway.

In the mid-1990s the Comprehensive Advanced Life Support (CALS) Program was created after a four-year collaborative effort that involved several Minnesota professional and academic entities to improve the emergency care in rural health care facilities.[1]

CALS is designed for all members of the health care team who deal with emergencies.[2] The CALS training consists of three components: (1) home study completed prior to participating in the formal courses; (2) a two-day interactive, scenario-based CALS provider course typically presented in rural hospitals; (3)

a one-day CALS benchmark skills lab that focuses on the skills to resuscitate a critically ill or injured patient. Providers are encouraged to attend in teams consisting of a team leader, usually a physician, and other facility staff.

Four thousand heath care providers have attended CALS since its inception in September 1996. The majority of courses have been held in Minnesota (160), in Wisconsin (6), and for the U.S. Department of State Medical Personnel who staff U.S. embassies around the globe (14). Several hundred CALS skills labs have been conducted in Minnesota and Wisconsin.

The real success of the CALS Program should be measured by the positive changes that occur in the care given to the seriously ill or injured patients who present to the doors of our rural hospitals. This is hard to measure, and to date no formal CALS outcome study has been conducted. We do have many anecdotal examples that suggest positive results. Helicopter-critical transport teams have noticed an improvement in patient airway management by hospitals that have participated in CALS training. The use of RSI (Rapid Sequence Intubation) in rural Minnesota hospitals has increased significantly. The success rate of performing rescue airway procedures has been very high among those trained with CALS. The time needed to stabilize trauma victims for transport has been reduced. Rural providers who have participated in a CALS course report having greater comfort levels when they encounter critical patients. Tertiary centers have noted an improvement in the condition of patients initially managed in rural hospitals.

Other states with large rural populations are interested in developing the CALS Program, which was originally developed and introduced in Minnesota. In response, a national CALS Program, incorporated as a 501(c)(3), has been organized to assist other states in this effort. The Minnesota State Trauma Advisory Council accepted CALS as one of the educational training programs to prepare level III and IV trauma center personnel for its institution's trauma designation. The U.S. State Department has designated CALS as its advanced life-support training program to prepare its medical personnel. Afri-CALS is being developed in Nairobi, Kenya, a version designed for the developing world with a different set of needs and resources.

CALS training offers an approach to the care of rural emergency patients and emphasizes teamwork. Team members learn a universal systematic approach to the critically ill and injured patients using basic, affordable, easy-to-use equipment. In the process, CALS also helps a rural hospital understand its limitations. According to one physician, "The philosophy of CALS is not that we, as a rural hospital, are going to be able to take care of all clinical situations on our own. Instead, the goal is to increase our ability to rapidly stabilize patients, rapidly determine their conditions, and rapidly transfer to appropriate care."

Notes

1. Under the initial umbrella of the Minnesota Academy of Family Physicians, the professional and academic entities involved were the Minnesota Chapter of the American College of Emergency Physicians, the University of Minnesota Department of Emergency Medicine, the Emergency Department of Hennepin County Medical Center, and the Department of Family Practice and Community Health at the University of Minnesota.

2. This includes physicians, nurses, physician assistants, nurse-practitioners, paramedics, nurse anesthetists, and other allied health care professionals who make up the team that deals with the emergencies rural providers confront in their emergency departments.

Blog: Rural Mississippi—
Aftermath of Hurricane Katrina

SHAILENDRA PRASAD

August 2005. I planned on flying back to New Orleans after a conference in Arizona. My wife and son had accompanied me. We watched Katrina grow like a weird reality show—a petulant child gaining weight, becoming unruly. There was talk about this being bigger than Ivan from the year before, even bigger than Camille from 1969. "No," my friends and patients in Mississippi told me, "nothing gets bigger than Camille."

Our flights home were canceled. Then we learned our neighborhood was under mandatory evacuation. Evacuation was not foreign to us. We'd participated in four drills during our seven years in Mississippi. "Hurricane parties," we called them. We'd lock the shutters on the house, secure the garage door, and remove the yard implements that could become missiles in the sixty plus mile-per-hour winds. Then along with our two satchels filled with a change of clothes, our son's favorite toys, and copies of our important documents we would drive to a safe home, a friend whose home was not in the path of the storm. We'd spend the night playing cards, talking, and waiting out the squall. Usually we could go home the following morning.

We hoped this, too, would pass and called a friend who had a spare key to our house.

"Sounds like a bad one," our friend said.

"Can you get our hurricane satchels? There are two of them, in the closet in the master bedroom."

"Sure. I'll lock up the house too. Anything else?"

"Yeah, put the birdfeeders in the garage. The birdbath too."

"Of course. Be safe. I'll be in touch."

That night in Phoenix I watched the television. Reporters talked about the rain and wind in surrounding areas. Counties in both Mississippi and Louisiana were evacuated. I called every number in my cell phone. No answer at the hospital, the clinic. My practice partner did not respond at his home phone or cell. I could not reach our neighbors or local friends.

Our county, Pearl River, and our town, Picayune, were orange on the weather map. The Internet news pages said nothing more. I could not eat dinner. I continued to make calls. I phoned my dozen sickest patients whose numbers I kept just in case they needed me. No one answered. I worried about my three-year-old patient waiting for a renal transplant at Tulane. He'd just gotten a match. What would happen now? No answer. And there was complicated Mr. Shirley who I just referred to the neurologic unit in Birmingham, Alabama. Would he get there for his appointment? When was that appointment? No answer. Then there was my dialysis patient. Where would she go? No answer. Feeling restless and helpless I walked down to the business center and opened this blog:

Pearl River County Katrina Survivors
This is my attempt to help in the aftermath of Katrina. I work in the Picayune area and have very dear friends in the area.
    The only precondition to this blog is this—respect your fellow bloggers. Please blog away to add on to the information on Picayune/Pearl River County, Mississippi.
posted by sprasad @ 8/30/2005 07:54:00PM

By midnight there were thirty posts. *I am looking for . . . I am trying to reach . . . does anyone have any information on . . .*
    Blogger Tom said:

I live outside of Picayune near Old Salem on Old Kiln Road.[1] I have my dog at the Picayune Vet clinic and I am worried sick. I did hear on CNN that downtown Picayune is starting to flood and government officials had to leave? I also heard from a co-worker that there is alot of wind damage. Let me know any info about picayune, the Vet's office and whether or not my dog is ok.
8/30/2005 08:11:00PM

Blogger Dave wrote:

I'm looking for some info on my son. His name is Danny Thompson and he had just moved to Picayune so you probably don't know him but you might know who he lives with. I'm sorry to say I only know her first name and it is Kathy (she's about 20 yrs old). They live on Salem Rd. Picayune, MS 39466
    I think her last name may be Sims or Fisher . . . confusing I know but we have little contact. I doubt you can do any good with this little info but I thought it was worth a try. Thanks for trying to help
8/30/2005 09:09:00PM

Blogger Samhanb said:

Can anyone tell me if the Heritage Inn has suffered any damage . . . I had several family members that evacuated from Slidell on Sunday . . . One of my uncles was sick and had to be taken from the hospital in Slidell. They all are staying at the Heritage Inn in Picayune. I'm in Calif and can't get through to anybody down there-thanks
8/30/2005 09:50:00PM

Blogger lookingforjoy wrote:

Can anyone help me with information about my Mother? My mother is Joy Parsons and lives in a remote area of Picayune. She lives on Hickory Road close to Chestnut Road. I talked with my brother yesterday and his family and house faired well. He lives in Ozona. I am very concerned and information is better than none.
8/30/2005 10:10:00PM

Over seventy messages were posted on August 31, 2005. I spent most of the day either glued to the television or checking the blog. Attempts to contact local friends and colleagues on my cell phone were for naught.
Sprasad said:

Samhanb:
I have found more postings on Slidell on the nola website under St. Tammany Parish -www.nola.com/forums/sttamtownhall/ you may want to try that blog.
8/31/2005 08:01:00AM

Blogger Tammy said:

The Delaney family has been found and are doing well. Thank you to the person who started this board. It has been most helpful! Thank God for answered prayers!
8/31/2005 10:09:00AM

Blogger John wrote:

lookingforjoy please email me with your email address as we are looking for people in the very same little neighborhood. Your mama's name sounds very familiar to me. thanks, John
john@mississippi.com
8/31/2005 11:08:00AM

Sprasad said:

Second hand information from Hide-away lake area. . . . lots of trees down . . . some structural damage to houses. No casualties reported. No power/no land lines. Bellsouth is working on land lines . . . so keep trying periodically. I59 closed from Hattiesburg south due to lots of trees down. Crews coming in from Jackson to clear it. May take ~48 hrs to clear it.
8/31/2005 12:51:00PM

Blogger Jones wrote:

Open Red Cross shelters. First Baptist Church of Picayune on Goodyear Boulevard. Roseland Park School in Picayune. Poplarville Middle School. First Baptist Church of Poplarville.
8/31/2005 01:00:00PM

Finally some footage from Mississippi was shown on television.
Blogger Frank said:

I have a few family members that was stuck in Picayune in a church not sure which one any info please help! ALSO my step father was on the highway last time I talked to him he was under an over pass by McNeal he could not go anywhere. His cell phone has gone out and no one has been able to find out info from Mississippi other than the coast and that is not right. The helicopters fly all over the coast showing video and that is as far as they are going. Do they not care about the parts of Mississippi that don't have the casino's where there big money makers are?????????
8/31/2005 01:52:00PM

Blogger Amy said:

PLEASE HELP. My sister is in Leakesville, Miss. its in Greene County. I am so worried about her, kids, brother in law and his family. No info is being given about anywhere around here. I have not talk to her in 3 days, i have not went to sleep yet been on the phones and online trying to find out something. If anyone knows info about that area PLEASE email me amy@mississippi.com. I know the house they were in before the storm hit is at this address: 321 Walnut St., Leakesville. PLEASE PLEASE HELP WITH ANY INFO
8/31/2005 02:10:00PM

Blogger Michelle said:

There's a news station out of Missouri who did a news report out of Picayune on the damage there. Here's the web address for the video footage and news report: www.ky3.com
I pray that everyone's families and friends are fine. I was born and raised in Picayune and still have most of my family there, so I have been worried sick. God bless you all!!!
8/31/2005 03:39:00PM

Blogger MSgirlnowMO wrote:

hi dr prasad. it's your patient Rose White. I found this from my family in TX. as you know I am in MO. i have spoken to mom monday evening after the storm passed. many trees down- one on our house- but mom, dad, Tony jr are o.k. i did not think to ask her about the hospital. I am trying to find out anything about Picayune especially Hideaway for mom's sis donna. They want to return, but from what i have heard it is not possible. Have you spoken to your wife and child? i hope all is well. email me at Rose@mississippi.net
    Rose
8/31/2005 03:42:00PM

Sprasad said:

Thanks Michelle for that footage from Missouri. Many have voiced concern that Picayune was not getting enough coverage. . . . I guess the devastation is mindboggling and it is not possible to get all the information across. Appreciate your input.
    Rose, hi. Good to know the family is doing good. Did you hear of anybody else . . . just blog all the names of people who are safe. It might help somebody. Yes my wife and kid are safe here with me. We were in Arizona for a conference prior to the evacuation. Desperately wanting to go back. . . . not able to.
8/31/2005 03:52:00PM

Blogger MSgirlnowMO said:

dr prasad (or anyone) . . . my aunt is wants to ask you some questions through me. #1 are they letting people into the picayune area #2 do u know of any passable roads to take from texas to ms? #3 do you know if ppl r working on power, water etc #4 i heard that the only place to get gas was in jackson . . . is that correct?

they are in TX and desperate to get back! from all accounts i have heard of and from ppl trying- i hear it is a good idea to stay put. is that true?

MSgirlnowMO (Rose)

8/31/2005 08:58:00PM

Sprasad said:

MSgirlnowMO/Rose

From MDOT they are not letting anybody but relief and emergency workers in to the Picayune area. Will let you know if I get to know anything else

8/31/2005 09:23:00PM

Blogger Tina wrote:

Dr Prasad my mom Florence is staying with me in New York. She is well but she needs her prescriptions refilled. I have made arrangements for her to see my family physician while she is here. The physician may have questions if you have a contact# where the Doc can reach you if needed please email me TinaA@ mississippi.com thanks for all the great work

8/31/2005 10:12:00PM

Blogger searchingforgrandma said:

I am in Guam. I am trying to find out anything I can about June Malloy. She lives on Elm Avenue in Picayune. If anyone has any information it would be greatly appreciated.

Jill

9/01/2005 10:01:00AM

Blogger Mel said:

I am currently living in Japan at Yokota Air Force base. I am trying to locate my family. They lived in Picayune, MS. My mother Thelma Travis, father Richard Travis, brother John, brother Gus

9/01/2005 10:12:00AM

Blogger anxiousSA said:

We are in South Africa and really need to know what has happened to our family in Picayune. Travis, Teri and Tom (11 years old) Walters from Oak street

Picayune. Teri used to volunteer at one of the vets. Please ANY info email us at Al@capetown.co.sa. Our prayers are with all those stuck in picayune and anxious families too.
9/01/2005 10:22:00AM

Blogger Washington said:

GOD BLESS YOU FOR THIS SITE, DR. PRASAD! I LIVE IN WASH-INGTON STATE AND HAVE A SON JACOB PERRY. THAT LIVE AT SYCAMORE DR. IN HIDEAWAY LAKE IN CARRIERE. HAVE HEARD NO NEWS THRU' THE MEDIA ON THIS AREA. DOES ANYONE KNOW OF THEM AND THEIR SAFETY. WHAT WAS THE DAMAGE IN THE AREA. THEY HAVE A BRICK HOME WITH LOTS OF TREES AROUND THEM. ANY NEWS WOULD BE APPRECIATED. HELEN 123-456-7890 (cell) helen@washinton.org
9/01/2005 11:53:00AM

Blogger MSgirlnowMO wrote:

INFORMATION FROM PICAYUNE as of 11:30AM THURSDAY
this is missouri girl again. i have talked to Bill (my dad) he was waiting in a mile long gas line in Hattiesburg ms (he says that there is like 2 places in the burg to get gas) he said that Crosby Hospital is still open and running. the beds on station one and two are all empty but I.C.U. is still running with people that work there sleeping there . . . including Dr. R. My mom worked last night and they did have 1 admit last night- for what i dunno.

dad went to hideaway lake it's pretty bad . . . but my aunt's house was virtually untouched in hideaway and they live on west lakeshore on the lake. so chances are your families are o.k. just structural damage. dad says some people are not being too friendly, getting annoyed with situation.

picayune no power no water . . . but there are various places set up around town to get ice water and military MRES [military meals ready to eat]. he said they have one station he knows of set up at claiborne hill. brother got MRE meals there. this is being set up by the great people of SPRINGFIELD MO (yay!) and in collaboration with the great people of Resurrection Life, who already do so much for the Picayune people.

dr. prasad--u were right . . . inherent good is in everyone . . . as i have learned from KS and witnessing all of this. (if you don't personally know the man that set up this blog . . . it's a shame cuz he's awesome).

that's all i can remember from the conversation with my dad and yes i

scribbled many notes! God bless and take care. maybe i will have more news
from picayune when i speak to my brother . . . who is on his way to memphis
from picayune now. . . .
love, missouri girl (rose)
9/01/2005 12:13:00PM

Blogger Jake said:

Dr. Prasad
    Thank you for this blog site. It has been a very long 4 days trying to get in-
formation about Picayune. I still haven't heard anything from my brother bob or
my mother Naomi at Willow Lane. I noticed that Ed is looking for his brother
at Cherry Drive which is down the street from my mother, any information on
either would be greatly appreciated. Thank you so much
    I know I speak for others, this is an admirable and very kind thing that you
have done. We just needed some kind of information.
9/01/2005 03:22:00PM

On September 1 there were almost two hundred posts. Strangers helped
strangers locate loved ones, shared other Internet sites for news, any news, and
helped long-distance relatives and friends find out what was happening in the
county. The blog took on a life of its own. The bloggers became community for
each other, angst was shared. That day, now two days after starting the blog I
found NASA photos of our neighborhood. I called my wife. "Kiran, I think this
is our house. Come look."
    "That's our street. Here's the nearby circle."
    "Yes. This is the Besh's, that is the Winn's," I pointed to the gray boxes. "And
this is us."
    "It looks okay."
    "I can't believe it. . . . it looks quiet, like a graveyard."
    We were supposed to fly Continental into New Orleans. Our car was parked
there, but no airline was flying into the area. When I wasn't on the blog, I was
on the phone trying to reach somewhere close to home. No flights to Baton
Rouge or Mobile. Nothing. Finally four days after the storm, I booked a flight
for the next day (September 3) to Jackson, Mississippi. I planned to rent a car
and drive the three and a half hours home. I'd see with my own eyes what had
happened and figure out how I could help. Kiran and our son would remain
behind for now.
    That night Jamie, a nurse I knew, phoned me. "I heard your clinic was wiped
out."

Chills crawled up my spine. Home probably okay, clinic wiped out. But her next words were like a buoy. "Will you help me set up a clinic? My brother has donated his church, Resurrection Life."

"Of course," I said almost dropping the phone. Now I had a focus for my return. Jamie had already started to gather resources: diapers, baby food, clothing. Her husband would pick me up in Jackson. I kissed my wife and son good-bye, not knowing when I would see them again and uncertain about what I would find on this journey. My blog family was supportive. Ms. Jill, my new friend from the blog, originally from Picayune was signing on from Guam, and she promised to take over the blog. I felt her maternal presence reassuring; the blog was in capable hands.

Jamie's husband picked me up on the highway outside the Jackson airport, which was packed with travelers like me, desperate to learn some news about home. "Indian man with a suitcase on the highway," he said as I opened the door to his truck. "I figured you must be Dr. Prasad."

The population of our town was 16,000. Picayune was on high ground, eighteen feet above sea level. Over the next few days, the number rose to 43,000 with refugees from Katrina.

Sprasad said:

Hi everybody:

In Picayune now!!! Overall Picayune fared much better than the coast. Power up in some areas-Woods, Millbrook, Parts around center of town, Goodyear etc. Phones up in many more areas. . . . I am at the free clinic . . . currently at the old Walmart building with Resurrection Church. Many businesses are opening . . . our clinic should also be open this week. The hospital is trying to get all cleaned up and started ASAP. FEMA is currently manning the ER. There is gas in Picayune at Walmart, Exxon and Shell on Memorial . . . long lines still present. . . . will try to keep everybody posted. We are getting a lot of people from New Orleans Louisiana . . . one tragic story after another . . .
9/06/2005 08:22:00AM

A Wal-Mart in a former life, Resurrection Church was spacious. We separated one large room into private areas for patient care with a combination of old modular furniture and bed sheets. Our separators reached to seven feet, creating visual privacy, but voices echoed across the room. I went to the Crosby Memorial Hospital pharmacy at Picayune and asked what they could give me. The chief nursing officer gave me lots of Bactrim, Ciprofloxacin, and Doxycycline. We were ready to open our doors.

Sprasad said:

Hi guys:

In Picayune. things are improving. Gas is available . . . long lines . . . power is coming back section by section. The hospital is being manned mainly by a DMAT [Disaster Medical Assistance Team] team out of South Florida. The hospital is hoping to be back and running by the end of next week. All hospital employees returning please contact Ms. Frank.

Picayune is getting a lot of evacuees from St. Bernard and New Orleans. The news from the gulf coast is not good. . . . looks like Picayune did OK considering the surrounding areas.

Dr. Hale is open in the am. Dr. Lorenzo and Pipers are also open for a couple of hours in the mornings till power comes back. Dentist Torres indicated that he would be opening up tomorrow . . .

I have sporadic access to the internet . . . will try to keep posting. I am at the Free clinic everyday for now.

9/07/2005 12:29:00PM

There was no electricity, but we had water and flush toilets. We worked during the hours of light. At dusk we had a generator that we used judiciously. The receptionist sat at a desk near the entrance to the room. She filled out an index card with the patient's name, city, and any allergies. A church from Missouri arrived with doctors and nurses. They became our pipeline for usable supplies. A new crew came every week bringing precious medications and skilled help. Truckloads of supplies began to arrive, some utterly useless. The truck I will never forget was the one from the East Coast filled with expired ventilator supplies. I opened a box from the stack to look inside. I should have heeded the warning on the box. The address said "To Haiti," and a bright red stamp read "Rejected." We had no ventilator.

"We can't use these," I said. "Don't have much storage space. Please take them back." The driver cursed me. We did not have enough nurses to sort through the truckloads that might contain one box of useful medications or equipment.

The patients kept coming, patiently standing in line and waiting their turn. At one point up to three doctors and six nurses provided patient care. Healthy patients were put to work in the drive-by supply room. We handed out gallons of water, diapers, canned vegetables, and bags of clothes. One afternoon, a middle-aged man sat in the chair waiting for me. I greeted him and asked how I could help.

"Can you get me these meds?" He handed me a long list.

I scanned his list, took a deep breath and asked, "Which organ was transplanted?"

"My heart."

"How long have you been without your meds?"

"One day."

I gulped. "I can get you prednisone, but that's about it."

He shook his head.

"Look you've invested, what, one million at least in your heart. Let's get you to Memphis or Birmingham. We can send you in an army truck." He was off to Memphis that evening.

Within the month there were 672 posts on the blog. Most were written during that first week when there was a communication vacuum. Now I skim through the blogs with an image of the different bloggers and the friendships we formed through the keyboard. But it took two years before I was ready to look at the messages. The memories seep in between the words. I can smell the dampness, feel my foot slip on the mud-coated sidewalk, feel nauseated with the amount of food in an MRE, and hear the desperation in the voices of loved ones. I remember the angry tone and glare from the truck driver with the vent supplies. Now when I teach a course on responding to medical emergencies I ask my students, "Who are you going to help on your mission? Be very clear with yourself about why you are going." I'll carry these events with me forever.

Notes

1. All names and addresses have been altered to protect the privacy of the individuals. In addition, blog entries have been edited as little as possible to preserve the original content.

The Dressing Change

TARA FRERKS

I glanced at the patient chart—there was only her name, Mrs. Friedrikson; her age, sixty-six; and the vitals, normal temperature and blood pressure. After knocking on the door, I entered the exam room. "Hi. I'm Tara, a medical student from the university, working with Dr. Brown. He asked me to talk with you and find out how we can help you." I shook hands with Mr. Friedrikson and touched Mrs. Friedrikson on her thin shoulder to avoid the bulky dressing on her right hand.

"I need my dressing changed," she said in a grandmotherly voice. She cradled her right hand in her lap and shielded it with her other hand and arm.

Mr. Friedrikson, a few strands of gray hair combed across his bald head, sat on the edge of his chair, tapping his left foot on the linoleum floor. "Do you know that you are the fifteenth contact we've made trying to find someone to help us?" He thrust a paper bag filled with dressing supplies into my hands.

I placed the bag on the counter and then settled onto a stool to listen. I enjoyed the independence and array of experiences I'd encountered in this small Minnesota community. I asked one open-ended question, "What can we do for you?" and the Friedrikson's story came pouring out.

A few months ago, they had retired to a house on one of the nearby lakes. They were new to this town and clinic. Helping her husband of forty plus years with a kitchen project, Mrs. Friedrikson had been trying to steady a two by four he was sawing. Her hand slipped and the blade of the circular saw sliced deep into the flesh and bones of her right hand. With blood soaking an old towel, they drove to the town's emergency room. The ER physician deemed that the injury was too complex for the local surgeon to repair. An air-ambulance transported her to a trauma center for microsurgery. "We were discharged home last week, and they told us to get checked up here within the week," Mr. Friedrikson said. "We couldn't find any clinic that would see us. Finally, we just went to the local emergency room this weekend. I have to tell you, the surgeon who changed the dressing was kind of nasty."

"Now Herbert," Mrs. Friedrikson said. "He was probably very busy."

I controlled my smile, I'd worked with that surgeon.

"My other problem is that they discovered that I have a heart problem so they did more tests. I have a big bruise here." Mrs. Friedrikson patted her right groin.

"They transfused her with four units of blood," Mr. Friedrikson added.

"Are you able to climb up on the exam table? We'll take a look."

Mr. Friedrikson assisted his wife and I steadied her as she turned around to situate herself on the table, the paper crackling as she settled in. "Can you lie down?" I asked and adjusted the pillow behind the patient's head. As I lifted the patient's blue denim skirt, I controlled my breath as I took in the patient's swollen yellow and green groin. I grabbed a paper sheet from the drawer, and covered her.

"Pretty ugly!" Mrs. Friedrikson said. "Usually I wear underwear. But I can't get the leg band of my panties over my leg!"

I touched the leg. It was tense, like the skin of an apple but not excessively warm. "Did they catheterize your heart?" I asked.

Mrs. Friedrikson nodded.

"Are you on antibiotics?"

"Keflex."

"I'll be right back. I need to check with Dr. Brown and tell him about you." I wanted to secure his permission to remove the hand dressing and to order some blood work.

At the nurses' station, Dr. Brown looked up from his chart to listen as I filled him in. He asked me if I was comfortable with what I was doing. I nodded.

I returned to the exam room with a second pillow. Mr. Friedrikson was standing near the table stroking his wife's cheek and forehead. "Dr. Brown told me to go ahead and remove the dressing. He'll come in to check on us."

Mr. Friedrikson retreated to a chair as I positioned Mrs. Friedrikson's hand on the pillow. She looked away, gazing at her husband. First, I removed the fiberglass splint. It was gray and smelled. Slowly I unwound the bulky dressing and marveled at how sloppily it had been wrapped. The thumb was enclosed completely and the fingertips were not visible. Wrapped this way, it was impossible to check color and circulation. Her hand was still caked with dried blood. I removed the blood congealed under her nails with a split tongue blade. I worked silently, occasionally nodding my head in recognition as the Friedriksons recounted more details from their nightmare.

The surgery had been done at a large trauma center, two hours away. When they returned home, they had talked with home care agencies, the county health department, and other physicians, trying to find someone to change the dressing and check a blood count. In desperation they'd gone to the local emergency room over the weekend; one of the nurses there had suggested they see Dr. Brown.

A knock on the door and Dr. Brown entered the room. He greeted the couple and asked me to review the patient's history. Resting the patient's hand on the pillow, I summarized the facts.

The husband interjected, "Couldn't find anyone to see us, fifteen attempts."

In his gentle manner, Dr. Brown apologized for the state of health care in the United States. "You got caught in the umbrella of surgical services," he said. "What this means is that your insurance paid the trauma surgeon to change your dressings when they paid him for your surgery. But I'm sure you don't want to drive two hours for a dressing change several times a week. We can't bill, but we'll take care of you." He examined the patient's hand. Did you take a pain pill before you came in?"

The patient shook her head.

"Better give you one."

Mr. Friedrikson ruffled through the paper sack and pulled out a bottle. "Hydrocodone," he said. Twisting off the cap, he poured a round white pill into his wife's good hand.

I filled a cup with water from the sink. Dr. Brown helped the patient sit up so she could swallow the pill.

After she lay back down, Dr. Brown examined the hematoma in her groin. "You've been through the mill." He shook his head and touched her shoulder. "This will heal, but it'll take awhile. How's your patience?" He asked me about her medications and whether I'd ordered a hemoglobin.

"Here's the medication list." The husband jumped out of his chair and handed Dr. Brown the paper.

Dr. Brown reviewed it. "Looks good. The lab will draw your blood before you leave and we'll call you with the result this afternoon." He directed me to clean and redress the wound. "Anything else?" he asked.

"We have an appointment with the trauma surgeon next week," Mr. Friedrikson said. "When should we see you?"

"See me the following week," Dr. Brown replied. "Tara, you're doing a fine job. Come get me if you have trouble." Nodding to the husband, he left the room, closing the door behind him.

As I worked, I listened as Mr. Friedrikson repeated some of the particulars of their story. It was clear that he was angrier than his wife, maybe feeling some guilt. He clearly had taken the lead in trying to secure help.

I washed off the remaining betadine and dried blood, then patted the patient's hand dry, careful not to hurt her. "Want to take a look before I wrap your hand?" I asked.

Mrs. Friedrikson emphatically shook her head.

Using supplies from their bag, I carefully placed Telfa (no-stick gauze) over the healing lacerations, then wound gauze around the fingers and thumb, wrapping the thumb separately and keeping the fingers visible to just below the nails. I'd watched many dressing changes, but this was the first I'd done on my own. I gained confidence as I worked.

Two hours after entering the clinic, I sent the couple on their way. They left with a neatly applied dressing and two hours of telling their story. Now more confident in my wound care, I realized that today I'd made a valuable contribution to Dr. Brown and the clinic team. As a medical student I had the luxury of spending time with patients, listening and talking and hearing every detail of their nightmare in a way that Dr. Brown could not. Now, my challenge over the next years of training is to learn how to demonstrate the same humanistic care in a more compact interval. And maybe with advocacy on my part, I might see a saner health care insurance system during my career.

Thank God for My Ass

THERESE ZINK

I am not referring to my backside, although I do have a well developed gluteus maximus due to my stocky German build and fifteen miles of running every week. My ass is Jimmy, a shy miniature donkey (think Shrek's pal) who has been the companion of my horse, Indy, on my twenty-acre farm for almost four years. Recently Jimmy saved my ass. Please pardon my crass language, but it is the truth.

At about eight one evening, my cell phone chimed as I was driving home. The local nursing home needed help with an elderly gentleman who had been admitted three days earlier. My partner had given him some furosemide late that afternoon for congestive heart failure, but Mr. Olson was still edematous and very short of breath. "The family is upset and wants me to do something," the nurse reported. "His hemoglobin is four and his potassium is six. Will you talk with the daughter?"

A hemoglobin this low would require a transfusion of several units of blood, and the potassium suggested kidney failure. "Sure," I responded. Not wanting to be the student who lost her homework, I said, "But I don't know him. Please read me his diagnoses and tell me what meds he's on."

It took the nurse several minutes to tick off the list, which included some dementia and repair of a thoracic aneurysm seven years ago.

"How old is he?" I asked wishing I was not the one on call.

"Eighty-eight," she informed me. "He's very sick. DNR-DNI. The family is pushing me to do something. The daughter is really upset."

As I drove in the darkness toward home, I took a deep breath and readjusted the phone next to my ear. My new challenge flashed like a neon sign—the distressed family of a new patient who I didn't know. "Any thoughts?" I asked the nurse.

"The daughter is a handful. Good luck."

"Put the daughter on," I said and prayed for inspiration.

"This is Janet," the voice said. "You know me. My husband and I borrowed your donkey for our church's Christmas nativity pageant."

I thanked God for the connection, some place to start this conversation. "Of course, Jimmy. That was a cold day." I said and remembered that the shepherds, kings, even Mary and Joseph, wore snowmobile suits under their cloth costumes. Thick Sorel boots peeked out beneath their flowing robes. Jimmy was insecure without his buddy, Indy. So this manger scene had had a horse and a donkey. Janet and her husband had given me the digital photos that I had cut and pasted into my Christmas letter to family and friends. "I am glad to talk with you again, but I am sorry about the circumstances. Tell me your understanding of what's going on with your Dad?"

Janet cleared her throat. "My mom cared for him at home for six years. He started having trouble walking two weeks ago, so I started coming every day to help her. We decided he needed more than we could do and looked for a nursing home. There was an opening here, so we moved him last Friday. He's gone downhill since."

I heard the frustration and recrimination in her voice: Why was he doing worse, not better at the nursing home?

"The nurses tell me he has a lot of fluid in his lungs," I said. "We can help him breathe easier."

"Can you help him get better?" Janet asked.

"He is very sick. I don't think he will recover from this. We could send him to the emergency room, but that would just be temporary and I think it would be very hard for him."

"Are you sure?"

"He is very sick," I reiterated. "The ER would probably want to admit him to the ICU." I explained his lab work. "Today we have options, but the question is what your dad wants and how what we do affects his quality of life."

"Is he dying?" she asked.

"Yes," I said. Of course Janet wanted to know when. I assured her that I didn't know. "This might take some time or it might happen quickly."

"Should I call in the family?"

I asked where they lived. All were out of town except for her mom, who could come in tonight if needed. I suggested that Janet tell her mom what I had told her and let her make the decision. "I can talk with her tonight if you want and I'll be at the nursing home in the morning." Luckily weekly rounds were tomorrow. The conversation with Janet lasted about twenty minutes. She seemed calmer when I asker her to hand the phone to the nurse. I gave orders for morphine and reviewed the furosemide orders. The nursing home did not bother me the rest of the night.

The next morning on rounds, Mrs. Olson was stretched out in a recliner covered with a quilt. Her handiwork, I suspected. I examined Mr. Olson who slept peacefully, the head of his bed elevated to a ninety-degree angle. He was also propped up with pillows, his hands and ankles were edematous; he was sleepy and did not have much to say. I reviewed his chart. His primary clinic had done a physical last week and drawn some blood. Based on yesterday's values his kidney function was much worse. No blood count was done, so with a hemoglobin of four and no obvious source of bleeding now, I guessed that he had been anemic for a while.

I asked Mrs. Olson to join me in the conference room. A plump and affable woman, she adjusted her eyeglasses and sat down at the table between the nurse and me. We were joined by a medical student who was shadowing me for the semester. "What did your daughter tell you?" I asked.

Mrs. Olson's explanation made it clear that Janet had understood what I'd said last evening. Aware of my tight chest, I collected myself as if I were about to guide my horse across a jump, my senses on high alert to read every nuance. Married for over fifty years, in the last decade Mr. Olson had overcome a number of "close calls" with his health. Seven years ago there was his thoracic aneurysm diagnosed at Mayo Clinic after they returned from vacation. "The doctor told us that it could have burst at any moment. If it had happened at the cabin, Roy would have died. We were just plain lucky." She shook her head. The smile lines around her eyes and mouth indicated the joy-filled life they'd had together. "The ache had bothered him for a few days. You know, he didn't really want that surgery. He was ready to go then."

I did the math in my head; for that surgery he was eighty-one.

"But we wanted him to have it, so he did." She explained his tough recovery. "In hindsight, he might not have done it."

We discussed that recovery would be very difficult this time. I explained how we would make him comfortable and suggested that we involve hospice. Mrs. Olson had considered being a hospice volunteer and agreed readily. "I am glad he is here. I could not have handled this at home," she wiped a tear from her eye. "He is ready to go."

I thought about the language we use for death, dancing around the actual word: move on, pass on, go, expire. "It sounds like he's had a good long life," I said and took her hand. I'd been doctoring long enough to see how patients often choose their time to die, waiting for a child to arrive from out of town, or dying when a loved one left the room, knowing it was too much for him to be present. Now that Roy Olson was in the nursing home, his dying process could accelerate. I assured Mrs. Olson that I would talk with Janet when she arrived. I called hospice and continued my rounds.

In her late thirties, Janet arrived after her chores. Her long blonde hair displayed her Scandinavian heritage. I shook her hand. Her grip was firm and the skin dry and tough, the hand of someone who worked outdoors. We'd last met at the nativity display. She was decorating the church while her husband and daughter tended to the manger scene.

We gathered in the conference room around the same table. "Good to see you again, Janet. What questions do you have?"

"I need to understand this. My siblings will ask me exactly what is happening." Her voice was like fingernails on a blackboard.

I braced myself and explained that Mr. Olson's organs were shutting down. I talked about the fluid backing up into his lungs because his heart wasn't pumping, the kidneys not filtering the toxins from his blood, the low hemoglobin not carrying much oxygen.

Janet sat forward, "But he has bounced back so many times before. Why not once more?"

I shoved my defensiveness away and tried to find the words to explain that too much was broken. Mrs. Olson was quiet as Janet grilled me and asked me to go through her father's chart with her. She fired questions about his rapid decline. I slowed my breath and focused on her, finding the patience to answer her questions.

"I am not a health professional, but I need to understand this," she said again. I ignored my watch and thought if I invest now, this would have a better outcome.

Janet sat back. Maybe I had repeated the details enough. Maybe I had finally said it in a way she could understand. Maybe it was because the hospice nurse joined us. Janet shifted from accuser to daughter. She thanked me and asked, "How's Jimmy?"

"He is fat and happy," I said. "He doesn't have to do anything but eat." I had just returned from a medical trip to Nicaragua where all donkeys were gaunt with thin coats. "In Nicaragua they'd call him *gordo.*"

We all laughed. I reassured them that I was as far as the phone and left them with the hospice nurse. Mrs. Olson trailed me out of the room.

In the hall she clutched my elbow and said, "This is very hard for Janet."

"It's hard to let go."

"They were very close. They farmed together."

The next evening when I was in the barn cleaning Jimmy's stall, I got a call from the nursing home. "Mr. Olson has died," the nurse said. "We need to have you sign cremation papers." They would fax them to me at home that evening. After shoving my cell phone into my pocket, I reached for Jimmy and rubbed him behind his ears, long and tan and trimmed with a line of black. His entire black mane stood upright like a punk rocker's haircut. I told him how much he had helped me the last forty-eight hours. Jimmy turned his rear end toward me, his favorite place to have scratched.

This selection was previously published in the *Journal of American Medical Association* 299:16 (2008): 1879–80.

Contributors

RICHARD M. BERLIN, MD, is a psychiatrist who has lived and practiced in the Berkshire Hills of western Massachusetts for twenty-five years. He is the author of a collection of poetry, *How JKF Killed My Father* (Pearl Editions, 2003) and two poetry chapbooks, *Code Blue* (Poetry Society of South Carolina, 1999) and *The Prophecy* (Pudding House Press, in press). He edited a collection of essays titled *Poets on Prozac: Mental Illness, Treatment, and the Creative Process* (Johns Hopkins University Press, 2008). An associate professor of psychiatry at University of Massachusetts Medical School, he enjoys gardening, riding his mountain bike, kayaking, and pruning his apple trees.

TOM BIBEY (pseudonym), MD, is a family physician who has practiced in rural North Carolina since 1984. In addition to caring for patients, he has a regular blog, Stories of the Bluegrass Music Road, where he posts twice weekly.

C. D. BRADLEY-JENNETT, MD, is a medicine and pediatrics physician who practices and teaches residents at Morehouse School of Medicine in Atlanta, Georgia. She has written poetry for over twenty years and wrote this poem as a medical student. Her work has been published in her undergraduate and medical school literary magazines. She is married with two children.

ERIK BRODT, MD, completed a family medicine residency in Seattle, Washington, and is now living in Madison Wisconsin with his fiancé Amanda. He is clinical faculty in the Department of Family Medicine at the University of Wisconsin and works as a hospitalist. He is also an itinerant/locums physician at the Iliuliuk Family Health Services in Unalaska, Alaska, during the height of crabbing and fishing seasons. The experience that inspired his piece occurred during his elective in the Rural Physician Associate Program at the University of Minnesota Medical School.

DARRELL L. CARTER, MD, is a rural family physician who has practiced in Granite Falls, Minnesota, since 1972. He is cofounder of the Comprehensive Advanced Life Support Program, currently serving as program director, and is a clinical professor in the Department of Family Medicine at the University of Minnesota. He has served as a preceptor for third-year medical students in the Rural Physician Associate Program for many years.

MITCHELL L. COHEN, MD, has practiced family medicine in rural Washington State for five years. Medical students and family medicine residents spend time at his office. He is an adjunct faculty member at the St. Peter Family Medicine Residency Program in Olympia, Washington, and on faculty at the University of Washington School of Medicine in the Department of Family Medicine. He has three kids, enjoys cooking, writes about the nonclinical aspects of medicine, and writes the blog Notes from the Country Doctor.

MAUREEN CONNOLLY, MD, is a physician who worked on the Navajo Nation in the 1990s. She now practices medicine in the Midwest and writes poetry and fiction. Her work has been published in *Hammers, Tomorrow, Ariel, After Hours, River Oak Review,* and the international anthologies *Freedom's Just Another Word* (Outrider Press, 1998) and *Earth Beneath, Sky Above* (Outrider Press, 2000), among others. She has read at numerous venues in the Chicago area, including Printers Row, Around the Coyote Arts Festival, and Guild Complex. Her awards include an Illinois Arts Council Award in prose, and a fiction fellowship from the Ragdale Foundation.

CESAR EMILIO ERCOLE, MD, wrote this during his Rural Physician Associate Program elective at the University of Minnesota Medical School. He plans to specialize in urology like his sister and father and is in residency in Florida.

LYLE FAGNAN, MD, is a family physician in the Department of Family Medicine at the Oregon Health and Science University, Portland, Oregon, and director of the Oregon Rural Practice-based Research Network.

KATHLEEN FARAH, MD, is a family physician who has practiced in rural western Wisconsin for over twenty-three years. She and her husband have four children and three granddaughters who provide lots of entertainment. She also likes to read and spend time outdoors.

HOLLY FARRIS is Appalachian and has worked as a volunteer caregiver, an autopsy assistant, restaurant baker, and beekeeper. Farris is the fifth generation of her family to live on their farm in the mountains of southwest Virginia. Her short fiction has appeared in journals as diverse as *The Greensboro Review, Lodestar Quarterly,* and *Frontiers*. She has been nominated twice for a Pushcart Prize and recently for a Lambda Literary Foundation Book Award.

ANTHONY FLEG, MD, was a medical student in North Carolina when he wrote this poem. He is now completing his family medicine residency in New Mexico and continues to write poetry about patients who inspire him.

TARA FRERKS, MD, has completed her residency at La Crosse Mayo Family Medicine Residency in Lacrosse, Wisconsin, and is pursuing a fellowship in sports medicine. A patient during her Rural Physician Associate Program elective inspired her piece.

JOSEPH GIBES, MD, is a family physician who now teaches and practices at the University of Chicago (North Shore) Family Medicine Residency Program. After receiving a BA in English and almost pursuing a career as an orchestral clarinetist, he attended medical school, married a farm girl, and practiced in rural southwest Wisconsin for eleven years. He and his wife Amy have three children.

DICK GORDON hosts the weekday interview program "The Story with Dick Gordon." Produced by North Carolina Public Radio and distributed by American Public Media, the show is based on stories and interviews largely chosen by listener input. The program debuted in February 2006 and was originally broadcast five times a week on North Carolina Public Radio and Minnesota Public Radio. In 2007, the program was broadcast nationally. Prior to "The Story," Dick Gordon hosted "The Connection" on WBUR in Boston from 2001 to 2005.

LORENCE GUTTERMAN, MD, is a retired hematologist/oncologist who worked in Columbus, Ohio, and consulted at hospitals in the surrounding small towns of central Ohio. He writes poetry and stories and has been published in several literary journals. Since moving with his wife to Connecticut four years ago to be closer to their children and grandchildren, he has been teaching creative writing to medical, nursing, and public health students in the Humanities in Medicine Program at Yale University School of Medicine. He also teaches creative writing at a prison. He is writing a book of poems about his childhood in eastern South Dakota.

GWEN WAGSTROM HALAAS, MD, MBA, is a family physician and Associate Dean for Academic and Faculty Affairs at University of North Dakota School of Medicine and Health Sciences. She was the director of the Rural Physician Associate Program at the University of Minnesota from 2004 to 2007.

PATRICIA J. HARMAN, CNM, MS, is a nurse-midwife, who practices with her husband Tom Harman, MD, at Partners in Women's Health Care in Morgantown West Virginia. She holds clinical appointments in both the School of Nursing and the School of Medicine at West Virginia University and is the author of *The Blue Cotton Gown: A Midwife's Memoir* (Beacon Press, 2008).

DONALD KOLLISCH, MD, is a family physician who practiced in rural New Hampshire for over twenty years and taught at Dartmouth Medical School. He writes fiction and is now a faculty member at the Sophie Davis School of Biomedical Education at the City College of New York.

EMILY KROENING, MD, is completing a family medicine residency in California. She was a medical student in the Rural Physician Associate Program at the University of Minnesota when this experience occurred.

Megan Wills Kullnat, MD, is completing her pediatric residency at Dartmouth-Hitchcock. Her piece was written during a rural rotation in medical school in Oregon.

ANN NEUSER LEDERER, RN, has been a certified hospice nurse for many years. She has lived and worked in Pennsylvania, Michigan, and Kentucky. Her poems and creative nonfiction have been published in a variety of creative writing journals such as *Kalliope, Diagram, Cross Connect, Brevity, Wind,* and *Diner.* Her work has also appeared in various anthologies and in the chapbooks *Approaching Freeze* (Foothills, 2003), *The Undifferentiated* (Pudding House, 2003), and *Weaning the Babies* (Pudding House, 2007). She has a number of professional publications as well and is the proud mother of a recent graduate of the University of Pennsylvania School of Medicine.

DAVID LOXTERKAMP, MD, is a family physician who has practiced in Belfast, Maine, for twenty-four years. His memoir, *A Measure of My Days: The Journal of a Country Doctor,* was published by the University Press of New England, 1997. His work as a family physician was the subject of a *Life Magazine* photo essay in 1998 and an NBC *Nightline* documentary in 2000. Writing is his favorite pastime, and he has authored numerous articles for professional and lay publications, including the *New England Journal of Medicine,* the *Journal of the American Medical Association,* the *British Medical Journal, America Magazine, Commonweal,* and the *Boston Globe Sunday Magazine.* He has contributed to two anthologies: *A Life in Medicine* (The New Press, 2002), edited by Robert Coles and Randy Testa, and *Professions of Faith* (Sheed & Ward, 2002), edited by James Martin and Jeremy Langford. At present, he is writing a book on his life in medicine. He is married to Lindsay, and they have two children.

DEBORAH LEE LUSKIN, PhD, is a regular commentator on Vermont Public Radio, an editorial columnist, book reviewer, freelance writer, and author of the novel *Into The Wilderness* (White River Press, 2010). As a visiting scholar for the Vermont Humanities Council, Luskin has facilitated literature-based humanities seminars as part of Humanities at the Heart of Healthcare, a nationwide literature-based seminar that allows health care workers to explore difficult issues in modern medicine outside the clinical setting. She writes about medicine for major medical centers, both as a translator of technical information for patient understanding and as a profiler of physicians and hospital services. She has taught writing to a wide variety of students of all ages and abilities, from Ivy League students at Columbia College in New York City to inmates at Southern State Correctional Facility in Springfield, Vermont. She lives with her husband, family physician Tim Shafer, and their three daughters in southern Vermont.

DAVID McRAY, MD, is a family physician and faculty member with a residency program in Texas. He practiced in rural eastern Tennessee for nineteen years. In 2008 he joined the faculty at John Peter Smith Hospital in Fort Worth, Texas, where he did his residency teaching surgical obstetrics and helping develop their international health track. He enjoys teaching, writing, and traveling with his wife and three almost-grown children.

JAMES MOLD, MD, MPH, is a family physician in the Department of Family and Preventive Medicine at the University of Oklahoma Health Sciences Center,

Oklahoma City, Oklahoma and president of the Oklahoma Physicians Resource/ Research Network.

ANN FLOREEN NIEDRINGHAUS, RN, MSW, wrote "Early Marriage" while making home visits as a public health nurse in a federal maternal and infant care program based in Morgantown, West Virginia. She is now retired and resides in Duluth, Minnesota, with her oncologist husband. She has written poetry for fifteen years and has had numerous poems published in journals and anthologies, including two chapbooks: *Life Suspended* (Poetry Harbor, 2003) and *Parallel to the Horizon* (Pudding House, 2007). Her work, along with that of four members of her longtime poetry group, is included in the anthology *The Moon Rolls Out of Our Mouths* (Calyx Press, 2005).

GODFREY ONIME, MD, is an internist in Lumberton, North Carolina. Twenty years ago, after high school in Nigeria, he immigrated to New York City. He completed his Bachelor's degree at Brooklyn College, medical school at the New York University, and residency training at the Presbyterian Hospital of the Columbia University Medical Center, all in New York City. After residency, he had a short stint practicing primary care in upstate New York, before moving to Durham, North Carolina to train in gastroenterology. However, he quickly realized that his passion was in primary care and "giving voice" to his patients through writing. He returned to primary care but chose to remain in North Carolina, settling in Lumberton, a region with a large proportion of Native Americans of the Lumbee tribe. He has practiced there for five years "as a boonies doc," according to his medical school colleagues in the Northeast. He is completing a book about the intersection of his background in Africa and his experiences in medicine in both the big and small cities of America.

WILLIAM OREM, MFA, PhD, worked for several years in a clinical psychobiology lab at the National Institute of Mental Health. His short stories and poems have appeared in over ninety-five journals including *The Princeton Arts Review, Sou'wester,* and *The New Formalist.* He has twice been nominated for the Pushcart Prize and won the Great Lakes Colleges New Writers Award, formerly given to Sherman Alexie, Louise Erdrich, Richard Ford, and Alice Munro. His collection of stories includes *Zombi, You My Love* (Questa Press, 1999) and *Across the River* (Texas Review Press, 2009). Currently he is writer-in-residence at Emerson College and writes a science blog.

MICHAEL PERRY is a nurse, emergency medical responder, and firefighter. He has written for *Esquire, The New York Times Magazine, Outside, Backpacker, Orion,* and Salon.com and is a contributing editor to *Men's Health.* His essays have been heard on National Public Radio's *All Things Considered,* and he has performed and produced two live audience recordings ("I Got It From the Cows" and "Never Stand Behind a Sneezing Cow"). His books include *Why They Killed Big Boy . . . and Other Stories* (Whistlers & Jugglers Press, 1996), *Off*

Main Street (Harper Perennial, 2005), *Population 485,* (Harper Perennial, 2007), *Truck: A Love Story* (Harper Perennial, 2007), and *Coop: A Year of Poultry, Pigs and Parenting* (Harper Collins, 2009).

SHAILENDRA PRASAD, MD, is a family physician who was educated in India and Detroit, Michigan. He practiced in rural Mississippi for nine years. In 2007, he left Mississippi to pursue an academic career in Minnesota. Now he teaches family medicine residents and does research in health policy to improve access and care in the rural United States.

MICHAEL R. ROSMANN, PhD, is a farmer, clinical psychologist and the executive director of AgriWellness, Inc., Harlan, Iowa, a nonprofit organization that provides behavioral health support for the agricultural population. He is an adjunct faculty member in the College of Public Health at the University of Iowa and lectures at many universities throughout the United States and other countries. He and his wife live in the farmhouse they built near Harlan. For the last thirty years he has devoted his life to working with and learning from farm and ranch people. He has been published in a wide variety of scholarly journals, literary magazines, and farm publications and has participated in National Public Radio, *National Geographic,* and television programs.

ARNE VAINIO, MD, is a family physician who went to medical school in Duluth and completed his family practice residency at the Seattle Indian Health Board and Providence Hospital in Seattle, Washington. Born to a Finnish father and a full-blood Ojibwe mother, he is an enrolled tribal member of the Mille Lacs Band of Ojibwe. Since 1997, he has practiced on the Fond du Lac Ojibwe Reservation in Cloquet, Minnesota, and teaches with the Duluth Family Medicine Residency. He writes articles for *News From Indian Country,* a national Native American newspaper.

ABRAHAM VERGHESE, MD, is an internist and infectious disease specialist and the author of many essays and stories published in both the lay and medical press, including the *New Yorker, The Atlantic,* and the *New York Times Magazine.* He is also the author of *The Tennis Partner* (Harper Perennial, 1999) and his most recent book, *Cutting for Stone* (Knopf, 2009). Currently he is a professor of medicine at Stanford University.

JOHN M. WESTFALL, MD, MPH, is a family physician in the Department of Family Medicine at the University of Colorado, Denver, and the director of the High Plains Research Network.

THERESE ZINK, MD, MPH, is a family physician who practices and lives in rural Minnesota, does research, and teaches in the Rural Physician Associate Program at the University of Minnesota. Her creative work has appeared in literary and medical journals such as the *Journal of American Medical Association.* She has completed a memoir on an international aid experience in Chechnya. An excerpt received a writing award from *Pilgrimage,* a creative writing/poetry journal in

Colorado. A collection of stories about doctoring and healing explores how the act of listening and holding stories is a vital part of healing for both the patients and the healer. One of these stories won the annual Medical Musings Writing Contest in *Minnesota Medicine* in June 2009. As a professor in the Department of Family Medicine and Community Health at the University of Minnesota, she works with medical students to write and publish the "interesting stories" that they post in online discussions or share during "significant event analysis" sessions.

Permissions and Acknowledgments

Cesar Emilio Ercole: "Pursuing the American Dream" appeared in *Minnesota Medicine,* February 2009. Reprinted by permission of *Minnesota Medicine.*

Holly Farris: "Cord" appeared in *Lockjaw: Collected Appalachian Stories* © 2007. Reprinted by permission of Gival Press.

Dick Gordon: "Robotic Docs" aired on "The Story," American Public Media, October 16, 2007. Reprinted by permission of North Carolina Public Radio.

Donald Kollisch: "Good Will" appeared in *Dartmouth Medical Magazine,* Summer 2000. Reprinted by permission of *Dartmouth Medicine Magazine.*

Emily Kroening: "Learning from an Amish Birth" appeared in *Family Medicine* 40:2 (February 2008). Reprinted by permission from the Society of Teachers of Family Medicine, www.stfm.org.

Megan Wills Kullnat: "Boundaries" appeared in *Journal of the American Medical Association* 297:4 (2007): 343–44. Copyright © 2007, American Medical Association. All rights reserved. Reprinted by permission of the American Medical Association.

David Loxterkamp: "A Vow of Connectedness: Views from the Road to Beaver's Farm" appeared in *Family Medicine* 33:4 (April 2001). Reprinted by permission from the Society of Teachers of Family Medicine, www.stfm.org.

Deborah Lee Luskin: "Mom and Pop Doc Shop" appeared as "Care Package" in *Dartmouth Medical Magazine,* Fall 2007. Reprinted by permission of *Dartmouth Medicine Magazine.*

Godfrey Onime: "When Hostility Melted for the 'Funny Accent'" appeared in *The New York Times,* May 27, 2008, © 2008 *The New York Times.* All rights reserved. Used by permission and protected by the Copyright Laws of the United States. The printing, copying, redistribution, or retransmission of the Material without express written permission is prohibited.

Michael Perry: "Call" appeared as pages 149–52 from chapter 9 of *Population: 485* by Michael Perry. Copyright © 2002 by Michael Perry. Reprinted by permission of HarperCollins Publishers.

Arne Vainio: "Mashkikiwinini: Thanking Sylvester for His Unconditional Smile" appeared in *News from Indian Country* (www.IndianCountryNews.com). Reprinted by permission of *News from Indian Country.*

About the Author

Therese Zink is a family physician
who practices in rural Minnesota
and is a faculty member of the Rural
Physician Associate Program at the
University of Minnesota Medical
School. She has written and published articles in medical journals,
contributed to books, served as
editor of a special issue on violence
in older women, and serves on the
editorial board of two medical/social
science journals.

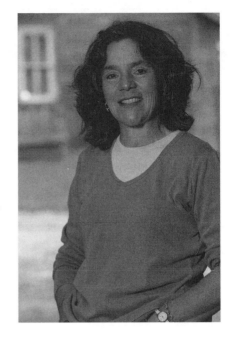

Literature and Medicine Series

Editors Carol Donley and Martin Kohn are cofounders of the Center for Literature, Medicine, and Biomedical Humanities at Hiram College. Since 1990 the center has brought humanities and the health-care professions together in mutually enriching interactions, including interdisciplinary courses, summer symposia, and the Literature and Medicine book series from The Kent State University Press.

The first three anthologies in the series grew out of courses in the Biomedical Humanities Program at Hiram. Then the series expanded to include original writing and edited collections by physicians, nurses, humanities scholars, and artists. The books in the series are designed to serve as resouces and texts for health-care education as well as for the general public.